M000025906

Acknowledgements

This project could not have happened without the tireless contributions and overall support of Catrin Schulte-Hillen. Séverine Caluwaerts also contributed hugely to this project. Several other members of MSF's Sexual and Reproductive Health Working Group provided invaluable guidance and contributions, including Eva Deplecker and Olivia Hill. Darin Portnoy and Greg Elder provided constructive reviews of all the material. Debbie Price and Meinie Nicolai provided particularly helpful contributions. Phil Zabriskie and Stephanie Davies contributed editing support. Communications officers in MSF offices around the world contributed material, including Sandra Smiley, Laura McCullagh, Vivian Lee, Yann Libessart, and Eddy McCall. Countless field and headquarters staff reviewed the material and provided important information.
Alexandra Brown, Doris Burtscher, Francoise Duroch, Atif Fazari, Asia Kamble, Marjie Middleton, Raquel Rosenberg and Karen Stewart provided early contributions. Meg Sheahan conceived of the idea that started this project.

All are warmly thanked.

New York, January 2015..M.P.

Table of Contents

Acknowledgements..5

Introduction by Meinie Nicolai..9

Chapter 1
Obstetric Emergencies: "If you cried here,
you'd cry every day"
By Séverine Caluwaerts..21

Stories from Patients and Staff...34

Chapter 2
Maternal Health Before and After Childbirth
Part 1: The Lead-Up To Birth: Essential Antenatal Care
By Nele Segers, with Olivia Hill and Eva Deplecker........................43

Part 2: The Risk Doesn't End When the Baby Is Born:
The Importance of Postnatal Care
By Debbie Price...52

Stories from Patients...64

Chapter 3
A Shameful Condition: Obstetric Fistulas
Contributions by Michiel Lekkerkerker...................................71

Stories from Patients...82

Chapter 4
"There is No Abortion Here" The Consequences
of Unsafe Abortion
By Séverine Caluwaerts, with Catrin Schulte-Hillen.............................93

Photo Stories
Saving Two Lives
By Martina Bacigalupo..105

A Second Chance
By Martina Bacigalupo..III

Delivering HIV-Free
By Sydelle Willow Smith..117

"Tari Women Are Very Strong"
By Kate Geraghty..127

No Good Choice
By Patrick Farrell...136

Chapter 5
Treating Sexual Violence: A Long-Term Commitment
Part 1: Women and Girls, Casualties of War
By Ann Van Haver...145

Part 2: A Scourge in "Stable" Places
By Rebecca M. Singer..153

Part 3: You Are Not Alone
By Aerlyn Pfeil...160

Stories from Patients...166

Chapter 6
The Evolution of Preventing Mother-to-Child Transmission of HIV
Part 1: Better Treatment, Same Challenges
By Helen Bygrave...179

Part 2: Whatever It Takes, We Should Do
By Pamela A. Onango 184

Part 3: A Shift in Thinking and Treating
By Joanne Cyr..188

Stories from Patients and Staff..194

Chapter 7
Breaking Down the Wall Between Maternal and Newborn Care
By Kristin Hooper, with Dr. Nicolas Peyraud.......................203

Stories from Patients and Staff..216

What It Takes To Make A Difference:
An OBGYN's Journal in Sierra Leone
By Betty R. Raney...222

The Contributors 240

Introduction

In 2006, I was part of an MSF team that was conducting an exploratory visit in Equateur Province, an isolated, underdeveloped area in northern Democratic Republic of Congo (DRC). One day, we visited a threadbare local hospital in a dusty village along the Congo River, where we were hoping to launch a medical response to a recent outbreak of sleeping sickness.

As I entered the facility, I saw a body lying on the floor, covered by a blanket.

"Did someone die?" I asked.

"Yes," I was told. "That is a young woman who died giving birth."

I never learned the young woman's name, but I've never forgotten her. I knew that health facilities in that area were desperately short of resources and trained health personnel. I knew that many women around the world don't have the power to make crucial decisions, such as whether or not to spend money to hire a vehicle to get themselves to the nearest hospital, even when they desperately need to go. And I knew the statistic that tells us that some 800 women die due to pregnancy-related causes every day.[i] But I also knew it did not have to be that way. And seeing her lying there, like an afterthought, hit me hard.

It also made me angry. As a nurse, seeing a woman die needlessly because she could not access medical care made me want to shout from the rooftops. That was years ago, but I'm still angry about it now, because deaths like these are happening with horrifying frequency to this day—and they can be prevented.

There has been progress in the realm of women's health. Between 1990 and 2010, there was a 45 percent drop in maternal mortality worldwide, according to the World Health Organization.[ii] The United Nations Millennium Development Goals adopted by the international community in 2000 further sought to reduce global pregnancy-related deaths by three quarters by 2015.

This is welcome news, to be sure. But in many countries where MSF works, a shocking number of women are still being lost. At present, 38 times as many women die in childbirth in Afghanistan as they do in the United Kingdom. Maternal mortality rates are 178 times higher in Central African Republic than in Japan, and 220 times higher in Chad than in Sweden.[iii]

MSF has demonstrated that it doesn't have to be this way, that simple, inexpensive interventions carried out by trained health staff could save many of the 800 women who die every day from pregnancy-related causes. To cite just one example: In 2012, the organization started ambulance referral systems in the districts of Kabezi in Burundi and Bo in Sierra Leone. These are countries with some of the world's highest rates of maternal mortality but very few hospitals or qualified medical workers.

Previously, complications during pregnancy were a likely death sentence for mother and baby alike. With the ambulance referral system, however, when a woman shows signs of complicated labor, the local health clinic can call for an ambulance. The ambulance arrives and takes the patient, escorted by a nurse or midwife, to a hospital where trained staff are on hand and surgical and blood transfusion services are available, for free, around the clock. The results have been dramatic: The maternal mortality rate in Kabezi dropped 74 percent; in Bo, it fell by 61 percent.[iv]

MSF is a medical humanitarian organization that works in roughly 70 countries to treat people who have been affected by conflict, natural disasters, disease, epidemics, severe privation, and long-term neglect. At root, our mission is to provide lifesaving medical care to those who cannot otherwise access it.

I've been with MSF for more than 20 years, first working as a nurse in the field, then running projects in several countries before becoming director of operations. I now serve as president of MSF's office in Belgium. While we are not specifically a women's health care organization, most of our patients are women and children. In project after project, I've seen our waiting rooms and wards full of pregnant women, women who've been injured or fallen ill, and women with their children. I've seen the lengths women will go to in order to care for their children, walking great distances in dangerous circumstances to make sure they get vaccinations and treatment, or risking everything, including rejection from their husbands, to prevent transmitting HIV to their unborn babies.

These are remarkably strong women and they are anything but victims. Many perform backbreaking labor in addition to running their households and caring for their children and other family members. During conflicts and other events that cause displacement, they often take on even more responsibility, frequently acting as the sole caretaker of their family members. Yet in spite of the huge burdens they shoulder, they rarely possess the power to decide when they themselves can get lifesaving care.

On the day I saw the young woman lying dead under a blanket in DRC, I reaffirmed a decision I had made early in my career to be one of the voices within MSF that pushes the organization to pay particular attention to the specific needs women have in the contexts where we work.

I am still one of those voices, and I'm glad to say I'm one of many, as you'll see in the pages that follow.

Put simply, women have distinct health risks that men do not have, and these risks must be attended to. Let's start with the obvious: women get pregnant and bear children. Worldwide, more than a third of all deliveries have complications, and 15 percent of all deliveries involve life-threatening complications likely to kill women if they cannot access emergency care. Globally, at least 287,000 women die during or shortly after childbirth every year.[v] Many could be saved by effective surgery, trained medical workers who recognized the severity of their condition, transfusion services, prompt transport to medical facilities or closer proximity to existing ones.

In far too many cases, these things are simply unavailable. My colleagues and I have lost count of the cases we know of in which women in labor could not find or afford a ride to the hospital, or a woman walked for hours or days while in labor only to learn that there was no doctor she could see until the following morning, if at all, or that she would be charged far more money than she could pull together to get the care she urgently needed.

The women and girls who manage to survive a life-threatening complication without emergency care, the so-called lucky ones, will usually lose their baby and may develop an obstetric fistula, which, while not immediately life-threatening, can have profound consequences for their health and future. Many women with fistulas not only carry the grief of a lost child; they also face rejection by their husbands, their families, and their communities.

When a woman does manage to deliver her baby successfully, the lack of sufficient newborn care in many places jeopardizes her child's ability to survive the first few weeks of life. A newborn's chances of survival are even slimmer if the birth was prolonged and complicated. In 2013, 2.8 million babies died before they were a month old, mostly due to asphyxia, infection, and pre-term or low birth weight complications.[vi] Again, access to properly trained medical workers and relatively basic care could have saved many of these children.

There are solutions. Good referral systems with ambulance services are one. Maternity waiting houses are another. In places where a woman lives far from the nearest hospital, she can spend the last weeks of her pregnancy in a house near a working hospital, alongside other pregnant women who can then count on getting the care they and their babies need when they give birth. That's exactly what MSF offers in Masisi, DRC, at a 70-bed maternity waiting house that is almost always filled to capacity. This is another simple intervention with profound consequences.

The challenges women contend with go beyond childbirth, of course. For a host of reasons, women are more vulnerable to contracting HIV and they struggle to get treatment if they do. They also bear the terrible burden of possibly passing the virus to their child.

Just growing up female can lead to health risks: In many countries, the custom of female genital mutilation (FGM) persists, affecting up to two million girls each year. FGM has no health benefits and is extremely painful and debilitating, with both immediate and lifelong health consequences.

In wartime, access to health care often declines, affecting everyone. For women, though, conflict results in even fewer options in maternal or pediatric care, or vaccinations for their children. Conflict also creates environments of rampant exploitation of women and girls and of rape used as a weapon. Displacement in general, whether due to economic necessity or man-made or natural disasters, leaves women and girls more vulnerable to sexual violence and trafficking.

In many of the places where MSF works, women have no access to birth control and little control over their sexual lives. If a woman has an unwanted pregnancy, there are very few options. If she carries the pregnancy to term, she could bear harsh social consequences. If she decides to seek an unsafe abortion, as millions of women with no access to safe abortion do every year, she risks severe injury, even death.

These issues and the suffering they bring about are not new or unknown, yet they still have not been adequately addressed. MSF tries to help as many people as we can; more often than we'd like, we are the only medical organization in the places where we work. In 2013, for instance, we assisted with more than 182,000 births, provided medical care for more than 11,000 survivors of sexual violence, and offered prevention of mother-to-child transmission care to nearly 16,000 mothers living with HIV and their babies.

We're the first to say, however, that many women are beyond our reach, that there are many services that we do not offer at present (such as treating breast cancer), and that there are policy and human rights debates we don't get involved in beyond the framework of our medical activities, such as the fight for women's rights.

At the same time, though, we do advocate for the people we treat. We call on the international and humanitarian communities—along with national governments and parties to conflict—to act when lives are at stake.

This book is part of that effort, part of the call to all involved and to all who care that more should be done to address the specific medical needs of women and girls around the world. It is a collection of first-hand accounts from MSF aid workers—midwives, OBGYNs, physicians, nurses, and counselors—who have treated women and girls in a host of different countries and contexts over the past two decades. Their stories illustrate how limited access to health care can have devastating consequences for women the world over. They also show the tremendous impact that care can have on an individual's life.

This is not an academic book, or a policy book, or an "aid" book. It's an attempt to bring together the views and experiences of people who've been in the field and who can articulate both the depth and scope of the needs that exist—along with the opportunities to provide meaningful assistance. It includes the voices of women describing their stories and obstacles in trying to get the care they need. And it's capped off by journal entries from an MSF OBGYN who encountered seemingly insurmountable challenges nearly every day of the six months she spent providing care for women in Sierra Leone. Despite the struggles, she saw clearly the impact her work had on the lives of her patients.

In early 2014, I visited an MSF project in Bangui, Central African Republic. The country was and still is, as of January 2015, in the midst of a conflict that has killed tens of thousands and driven around one million people—20 percent of the population—from their homes.

At the Bangui airport, MSF has a makeshift field hospital next to a refugee camp where huge throngs are seeking sanctuary. We provide health services and emergency first aid, as we've done in many places over the years. But we also have a delivery room and a space to treat survivors of sexual violence. These, too, are an integral part of MSF's response. Bullets are often fired over the clinic and our staff members have to lie down until the shooting stops. But we have no plans to stop providing a space for women's health.

These women will not be afterthoughts. They cannot be, because, as the title of this book says, tomorrow needs them.

This is true in Afghanistan, Pakistan, Sierra Leone, Burundi, Colombia, South Sudan, DRC, and in every other country where MSF works—in every other country, period. As an organization, we look forward to the day when women the world over have access to the kind of medical care many of us in the developed world take for granted; to a future where no girl or woman has to die because she could not reach a hospital in time; and to the day when I can be confident of entering a remote rural hospital without seeing the body, shrouded on the floor, of a woman lost in childbirth.

I hope this small project goes some way to furthering this dream. And I thank you for your interest in the global crisis of access to medical care for women and girls.

Meinie Nicolai
President, MSF Belgium

[i] WHO, Maternal Mortality Fact Sheet, No. 348. May 2014. http://www.who.int/mediacentre/factsheets/fs348/en/

[ii] Ibid.

[iii] WHO, UNICEF, UNFPA, The World Bank, and the United Nations Population Division. "Trends in Maternal Mortality: 1990 to 2013," p. 31-35. 2014. http://apps.who.int/iris/bitstream/10665/112682/2/9789241507226_eng.pdf

[iv] MSF, "Safe Delivery: Reducing Maternal Mortality in Sierra Leone and Burundi," November 2012. http://www.doctorswithoutborders.org/sites/usa/files/MSF%20Safe%20Delivery%20ENG.pdf

[v] WHO, UNICEF, UNFPA, The World Bank, "Trends in Maternal Mortality: 1990-2010," p. 1, 2012. http://reliefweb.int/sites/reliefweb.int/files/resources/Full_Report_3984.pdf

[vi] UNICEF, "Child Survival: Neonatal Mortality Rates Are Declining in All Regions, But More Slowly in Sub-Saharan Africa," updated November 2014. http://data.unicef.org/child-mortality/neonatal

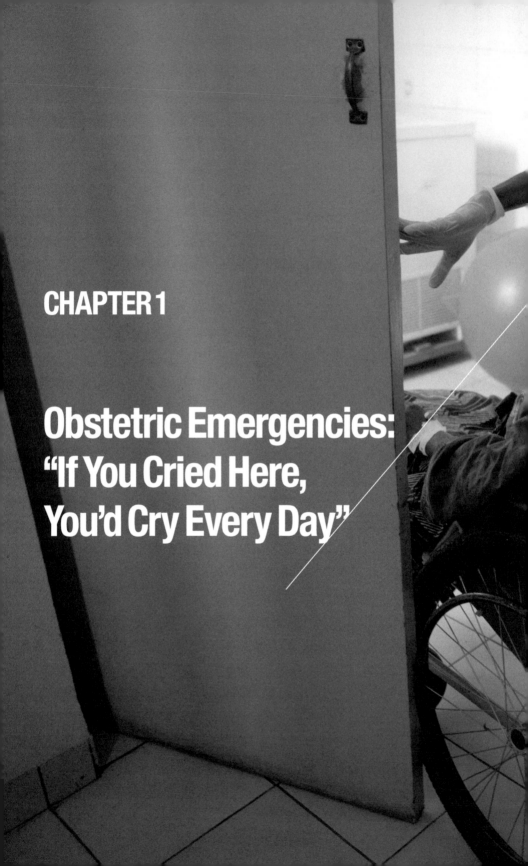

CHAPTER 1

Obstetric Emergencies: "If You Cried Here, You'd Cry Every Day"

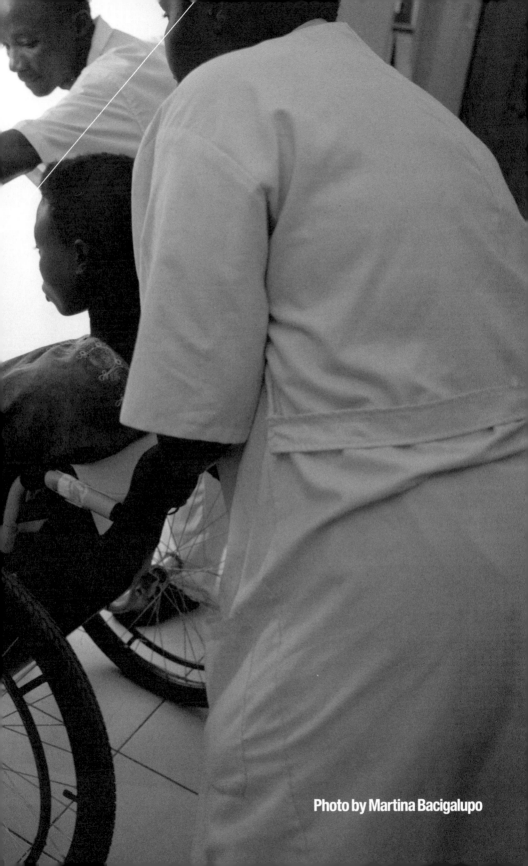

Photo by Martina Bacigalupo

Chapter 1
Obstetric Emergencies:
"If you cried here, you'd cry every day"

By Séverine Caluwaerts, OBGYN, MPH

MARIAMA

I had been the gynecologist at MSF's Gondama Referral Center in
Bo, Sierra Leone, for one month when a 16-year-old named Mariama
arrived at our clinic sandwiched between her mother and father on a
motorcycle. She was heavily pregnant, pale, bleeding, and in a lot
of pain.

Two nurses helped her off the motorcycle and put her on a stretcher.
One inserted an IV line while I palpated her abdomen and asked her
family what had happened.

Four days earlier, they told me, Mariama had gone into labor. Just as
half of all women in the developing world do, she tried to deliver without the help of a skilled health worker.[i] She was assisted by a traditional
birth attendant (TBA), who came to her home, but things did not go
well, and after three days, the family decided to come to the hospital.

It was the rainy season, however, which made a long journey even
more difficult. They had to travel the first leg by boat just to reach the
motorbike. The entire trip took a full day.

I had worked as an OBGYN in Belgium for ten years but this was my
first assignment with MSF, and I had never seen a patient in this state.
I didn't understand why the family would have waited so long to bring
Mariama to the hospital.

I came to learn that in this community everyone tries to deliver at home with a TBA. That's the custom. The problem is that most TBAs are not trained to identify pregnancy-related complications that require emergency care. Even when the complications become glaringly obvious, few families in this part of Sierra Leone—or in most of the country, in fact—can easily access a health facility with personnel trained to deal with such things. That is why pregnant women in trouble often arrived at our hospital in very advanced stages of distress. Some arrived too late to assist. Others never made it at all, dying en route.

I can't tell you the number of times I saw a patient in Sierra Leone or on subsequent MSF assignments and thought: "If only I could have seen this woman just a few hours or a day earlier, this disaster would not have happened."

Every day, in fact, about 800 women around the world die from causes related to pregnancy and childbirth.[ii] The majority bleed to death, succumb to severe infection, fall victim to a sudden spike in blood pressure (pre-eclampsia), or die after seeking an unsafe abortion. These deaths could easily be prevented with treatment that is not terribly complicated, if trained medical personnel and proper medical materials are accessible.

MSF teams assisted in 182,234 deliveries in 2013.

But in too many places it is not available, which is why MSF makes obstetric care a priority, running 131 projects with dedicated emergency obstetric services in places where national health systems are non-existent or have been severely affected by conflict or neglect. Obstetric care is also incorporated into nearly all MSF projects in conflict settings and other situations where large numbers of people have been cut off from care. Where necessary and feasible, teams provide surgical services as well. And they manage pre- and postnatal complications, along with problems resulting from unsafe abortion and miscarriage.

I have been on ten assignments with MSF in sub-Saharan Africa and Central Asia and seen far too many situations like Mariama's. The lack of access to emergency obstetric care is a problem that goes far beyond Sierra Leone, but Sierra Leone has long had one of the highest maternal mortality rates in the world—it had the highest rate in 2013, with 1,100 deaths for every 100,000 live births.[iii] It's no great mystery why: in Bo's government hospital, for example, there are almost no doctors, nurses, drugs, and hygiene.

It's heartbreaking. And our job is to assist those we can. In Mariama's case, we were quite certain that her uterus had ruptured during her prolonged labor. After the nurses and I rushed her into the operating room, I used a mixture of English and the local language, Krio, to explain to her parents that this was serious, that the baby was probably dead—very few babies survive uterine rupture that occurs outside a hospital—and that I would not remove Mariama's uterus if at all possible. But I needed their permission to remove it if it was necessary to save her life, I added. Her mother started to cry.

The baby was palpable inside the abdomen and was indeed dead, as the fetal heart monitor confirmed. We performed a midline laparotomy, opening her belly from above her umbilicus towards her pubic bone, and extracted the perfectly formed dead baby by his feet. Then came the effort to repair the rupture of her uterus, which extended all the way into her bladder. Were she still at home, she would have died within hours.

After this difficult surgery and a transfusion of three units of blood, we were able to stabilize Mariama. We had also been able to save her uterus, which is extremely important for a young woman in this context. But she was not clear yet. The baby's head had been pressing against her pelvic bone for so long that she had sustained a fistula—an opening in the pelvic tissue between her uterus and bladder. While not immediately life threatening, a fistula can cause significant and long-lasting physical and social problems for a woman. The sooner it was diagnosed and repaired, the better. When she was ready, we sent her to the nearby West Africa Fistula Foundation for fistula repair surgery.

In my first week in Sierra Leone, I performed four Caesarean sections in a row, all on pregnant women who came to the hospital long after they began experiencing serious complications. None of their babies survived; two died before the mother reached the hospital. In Belgium, I'd likely have tears in my eyes if a mother delivered a dead baby, in part because it happens so rarely. In Sierra Leone, I cried in the beginning, too. But it eventually became impossible to cry over every time— not because it wasn't just as tragic, but because I'd have been crying every day.

I was grateful when I performed a fifth Caesarean and out came a healthy little girl, alive and well. After the surgery, I took her in my arms and she started sucking on my finger, looking for milk. I looked at this beautiful, perfect baby and smiled in sheer relief.

Once, a mother arrived in labor, trying to deliver twins. She was from Bonthe Island—two days travel from the MSF hospital. Two men had carried her part of the way. Then she rode in a boat, then a private taxi. She urgently needed a Caesarean so we put her on the operating table right away.

The first of the twins was positioned with his chin, rather than the back of his head, pointing downwards. It was extremely difficult to extract him because he was stuck in the mother's pelvis, and when he came out he was not breathing. Our pediatrician tried to resuscitate him, to no avail. Luckily, the second twin was still breathing and was delivered successfully. That was a relief but it was gutting to think that the first twin died solely because his mother could not access transportation to the hospital in time.

This is something I saw in numerous other locations where I worked, including in Khost, Afghanistan. There, insecurity in the surrounding area prevented us from getting out on the roads ourselves, but in some places we are able to help bring women closer to care. In the Bo district of Sierra Leone and the Kabezi district of Burundi we started an ambulance service where a nurse or midwife accompanies the patient from a local clinic to MSF's hospital, giving her the drugs and fluids she needs during transportation. As a result of this system and the quality of care we provided, maternal mortality went down 61 percent in Bo and 74 percent in Kabezi between the late 1990s and 2012.[iv] It is hard proof of what can be done, and how many lives can be saved, with some relatively simple efforts.

ZOHRA

In January 2013, a pregnant woman named Zohra came to the MSF maternity hospital in Khost, Afghanistan. She was 34 and had already given birth to 11 children, nine of whom were still alive. When she got to the hospital, she was already bleeding profusely.

At that point in her life, Zohra had known that getting pregnant again was a health risk. But contraception in Afghanistan is difficult to obtain outside of the capital (and even in Kabul, it's not simple). Many women in Afghanistan live almost all of their lives at home, with no income of their own and little or no access to family planning. When the Taliban was in power, family planning was explicitly forbidden, and religious opposition to contraception runs deep to this day.

This has serious consequences. Studies by the World Health Organization have shown that providing contraceptive services has the potential to reduce maternal mortality by more than 30 percent, in large part by giving women more autonomy over their own bodies.[v] Yet access to contraception, including condoms, is very limited for many women for societal and financial reasons. The family planning services that are available where MSF works usually focus on postnatal birth spacing, and staff at the facilities often disapprove of sex outside of marriage. Many young women are alone when it comes to preventing and dealing with unwanted pregnancy. That is why providing contraceptives upon request to women and girls of reproductive age is an important component of MSF's efforts to prevent maternal mortality.

Before opening the hospital in Khost, MSF had arranged meetings with the religious leaders in the area and held several gatherings with community elders. What we heard gave us hope. Many of the community leaders had seen or heard about women dying in childbirth and they wanted to save their wives and daughters from the same fate, so they were very much in favor of MSF opening a women's hospital. They even allowed us to provide contraception, in the form of birth control pills and injections.

Zohra's case illustrated in fine relief the need for MSF's emergency obstetric services. Women like her who have borne many children face two main threats: first, repeated pregnancies stretch the muscle of the uterus to the point that it cannot contract adequately and thus cannot prevent dangerous, heavy bleeding. What's more, the muscle of the uterus may no longer be strong enough to move the baby into a good birthing position, making it more likely that a woman will have a complicated delivery. In addition, in women who have had previous Caesareans and those who have had several previous births, the placenta can attach to the uterine wall in an abnormal place and obstruct delivery. The potential consequences of each of these factors include severe hemorrhaging, uterine rupture, and death.

Before reaching us, she had made two prenatal care visits to a government-run clinic in her village. She'd also had two previous episodes of bleeding during this pregnancy. Still, Zohra assumed she would have her baby at home. That's how she'd delivered her previous children, after all. And it wasn't crazy to think doing so could be safer.

In Afghanistan, there are major difficulties with a hospital delivery. To start, the ongoing conflict can make it very risky to travel to the hospital. Local nurses also told me that some men in rural Afghanistan societies view women as not worth the resources required for a hospital delivery. The hospitals themselves are often under-equipped as well—the clinic Zohra had visited earlier did not have an ultrasound device, for instance.

By the time she reached us, Zohra had been bleeding heavily for two or three hours. Her baby was still alive, however. Through ultrasound we diagnosed placenta previa—the placenta was attached too low on the uterine wall, obscuring the opening to the cervix. This makes it impossible for the baby to move into the birth canal. What's more, every time the mother has a contraction, the baby pushes on the placenta. This is why Zohra was bleeding heavily.

We took her to the operating room and performed a Caesarean section. Her baby, a boy, survived, but Zohra's uterus did not contract as we'd hoped it would. She continued bleeding during surgery, and we needed to perform a postpartum hysterectomy—removing the uterus to stop the bleeding and save her life.

If MSF had not been there, Zohra most likely would not have gotten the Caesarean, let alone the hysterectomy. Her family was extremely poor and couldn't afford the cost of such a procedure in a government hospital. Zohra also arrived in Khost at night, desperate for assistance. In many government-run facilities with staff shortages, patients arriving overnight often are not seen until the morning.

Zohra needed four units of blood right away. They were difficult to get. We had to convince the family to summon men to donate blood, which was tricky both because of a cultural resistance to giving blood and the fact that no one wanted to drive to the hospital at night due to the conflict. I spent 30 minutes talking to her husband outside in the freezing Afghanistan winter, explaining how dire Zohra's situation was. He eventually agreed to call other family members to donate blood for his wife.

The issues around blood go beyond Afghanistan. In Sierra Leone, Mariama had likewise needed donated blood—three units in her case.

Her parents were willing to donate for her, but it was often a struggle in that country as well. There were all sorts of rumors about blood donation; I heard, for instance, that you drop dead the fifth day after donating or that it causes sexual impotence in men. I even heard people say they would not donate blood because MSF was selling it for a profit. This was nonsense, but I was still shocked.

It's with these sorts of concerns in mind that MSF tries to organize a blood bank in every hospital where we work. In Sierra Leone, our lab technician organized a one-Saturday-a-month blood donation day. We advertised on the local radio station and offered free food as an enticement. It worked to a degree, but for patients with rare blood groups, finding their types posed many problems. Blood can only be kept in the refrigerator for three weeks, and donations are needed continuously to ensure an emergency supply. In Khost, we eventually got the blood and Zohra recovered without complications. After one week she went back to her family.

RAZIA

It's not every day that a woman arrives at the hospital having delivered one baby two days earlier and with a second still in the womb, but it happened in 2012 while I was working in the town of Timurgara in Lower Dir, a mountainous district in northern Pakistan near the Afghan border.

Family members brought Razia by car over narrow, snow-covered roads from Upper Dir. It was January, a time when snow made travel in the area even more laborious than it usually was. Razia was 28. She had given birth to three children previously, but always at home, and that had been the plan again this time. It had never occurred to her husband and family to go to the hospital. Razia had sought antenatal care locally, but no one was able to tell her that she was carrying twins. After Razia delivered a healthy boy at home, she was stunned to learn that there was another baby inside her. More troubling was the discovery that the baby was in a transverse position, its umbilical cord already out. The family and the traditional birth attendant waited and waited, but the baby did not shift into a good birthing position.

At first, as religious people, they had faith that the problem would be resolved. But as time went on, they realized they needed help. Two days after she first went into labor, Razia's husband took her to the local clinic, which immediately referred her to MSF's hospital in Lower Dir. It was a big psychological step for them to leave their village for an unknown town, not knowing what to expect from health services in another region, not to mention driving along treacherous roads in a snowstorm in a war zone. But they were willing to go.

At the time, MSF was not organizing transport at night because of poor security, so Razia's family had to find their own way to the hospital. They arrived at two in the morning. Razia was stable and alert. To my surprise, the baby was still alive and its heartbeat was strong and regular. I performed an emergency Caesarean section and a screaming, healthy little girl was delivered. Our operating staff called her "a miracle of Allah."

Razia recovered quickly and was determined to get back on her feet the day after her surgery so that she could care for her new babies, and she left the hospital after five days. Before she departed, we offered her contraception, which would enable her to wait at least two years before her next pregnancy. She declined. Her two eldest children were girls, and she only had one live boy. There is a strong preference for boys in Pashtun culture, and she was hoping to have another boy soon. If she did not produce one, she worried she would not count in the eyes of her husband and her mother-in-law.

Razia and her baby girl were very lucky. The nurse in their local health care center knew about the MSF hospital. The MSF team upon arrival had organized meetings with the community in Timurgara to let people know that MSF provided lifesaving care 24 hours a day, seven days a week. But Razia was not out of danger. She now had a Caesarean scar, which put her at higher risk of complications during her next pregnancy. There were medical reasons that she should wait two years before getting pregnant, as we informed her. The scar may not be completely healed by the next time she tries to deliver.

I told her that if she became pregnant again, she would need to deliver in hospital. I'm sure she heard the message, which our local nurse translated to Pashtu. But I'm not sure she will follow our advice or that her husband will let her deliver in hospital, short of the emergency situation that brought her to us in the first place. If she did get pregnant again, I'd be worried about a possible uterine rupture, especially because she lives in a remote area, far from health care. This is why in places where there are few opportunities for a pregnant woman to find surgical care, MSF will only perform a Caesarean section on a patient whose life is at risk.

What strikes me about Razia's story, and that of Mariama and Zohra, is that I will never know what happened next for them. We met them at a moment of crisis, we solved a life-threatening problem, gave them advice for the future, then let them go. But anything can happen once they leave the hospital, and we can never count on them coming back, or being allowed to come back, the next time they need medical help.

If women in developing countries had accessible obstetric care in their communities, I wouldn't have to worry about Razia, Mariama, Zohra, and the hundreds of women I've treated over the years. Eight hundred women would not die every day while we know how to save them. It is tragic that in many parts of the world today, women have no access to quality obstetric care administered by properly trained staff.

Governments must recognize the need to provide emergency obstetric care for their citizens, and if they can't, for whatever reason, the international community must try to step in and provide those services. Even in conflict settings—especially in conflict settings—we have to find a way to attract doctors, nurses and midwives, and to make services available 24 hours a day, seven days a week, and to make transportation available as well.

Many nongovernmental organizations lack the capacity to provide hospital services and big donors—donor countries and organizations— are often reluctant to invest in them. But if we truly want to improve maternal mortality rates, they will have to find a way.

At MSF, we continue working to improve our quality of care in obstetrics, dedicating some programs exclusively to emergency obstetric care and integrating it in all our programs. We urge others in the international medical field and local health authorities to put the needs of pregnant women and their unborn children at the forefront of their programming. There are 800 lives (at least) at stake every day.

i UNICEF, "Maternal and Newborn Health," June 2012. http://www.unicef.org/health/index_maternalhealth.html

ii WHO, "Trends in Maternal Mortality," Fact Sheet No. 348, updated May 2014. http://www.who.int/mediacentre/factsheets/fs348/en/

iii WHO, UNICEF, UNFPA, The World Bank, and the United Nations Population Division, "Trends in Maternal Mortality, 1990-2013," World Health Organization, 2014. http://apps.who.int/iris/bitstream/10665/112682/2/9789241507226_eng.pdf?ua=1

iv MSF, "Safe Delivery: Reducing Maternal Mortality in Sierra Leone and Burundi," November 2012. http://reliefweb.int/sites/reliefweb.int/files/resources/MSF%20Safe%20Delivery%20ENG.pdf

v John Cleland, Stan Bernstein, Alex Ezeh, Anibal Faundes, Anna Glasier, and Jolene Innis, "Family Planning, The Unfinished Agenda," World Health Organization, 2006. http://www.who.int/reproductivehealth/publications/general/lancet_3.pdf

STORIES FROM PATIENTS AND STAFF

Bibi, 60, Afghanistan

"My daughters and my daughters-in-law deliver at home most of the time. If there are complications, they will go to MSF's Ahmad Shah Baba Hospital (in Kabul). My daughter just delivered a baby 15 days ago at the hospital. She felt such pain and she was very weak. We sent her by taxi. The transport fare was 200 afghanis [$3.50]. But when she arrived to the hospital she was not ready to deliver and she was sent back home. *[Note: MSF's hospital operates at full capacity every day and can only accept women ready to deliver.]* A few hours later, at midnight, she was ready to give birth and had to go to the hospital again, but we didn't have a car to send her. We knocked on the doors of our neighbors' homes because some of the families have cars. And finally we found someone to bring her to the hospital. It was not easy."

Rosaline, Bo, Sierra Leone

Note: This testimony was told two days after Rosaline's daughter-in-law was admitted with post-partum hemorrhage to MSF's Gondama Referral Hospital in Bo.

"At about 9 o'clock on Friday evening I was asleep when [my daughter-in-law] woke me. When I got up she said she was really feeling pain and could not bear it, so I took her to the government hospital. There was no nurse there during the night, so we slept and at 1 p.m. the next day she gave birth. After that she was bleeding, bleeding, bleeding. The doctor told us we could either take her to Freetown, or Mageni, or to Gondama hospital.

Straight away the nurses told us to go to the MSF hospital in Gondama. Luckily we have a car. She needed blood but we could not find anyone to donate. It was very late, so the staff found her two units of blood. If they had not, she would have died. I'm telling you the truth.

They told me that they do everything for the patient except provide blood—the family has to find blood themselves. If you come with people who donate it's OK. But if there is no one, the staff will try to find blood for you. And, indeed, they did for me. Right now we are still scrambling for more blood.

Parents have to go out by all possible means to find the blood. This morning I went as far as the junction. There I met some boys and we came back here together. Unfortunately, the boys' blood types did not match with my daughter-in-law. When my husband came with his brother, they also helped and we found someone who matched her blood type. We still need one more pint."

Ayak, 25, at MSF's Aweil hospital, South Sudan

"This was my third baby. The first two children are also not alive. When I fall sick in the village I usually come to the hospital, but it is very far. It can take one day on foot to come to the town because there is no health center nearby. I was brought to the hospital today by bicycle because I tried to deliver at home and the baby didn't come out. It took two and a half hours to arrive here by bicycle.

The labor pain came during the night, around 10 p.m., and lasted into the morning. My family had called the traditional birth attendant. She tried to help me but failed. Around 11 a.m., when we saw the baby was not going to come out, I came to the hospital. It was my uncle who decided I should go.

When I arrived here today the midwife tried to have me deliver vaginally but I was not wide enough, so they cut *[The staff performed an episiotomy]* in order for the child to be delivered.

With my two first children, when I tried to deliver at home, it happened the same way. There was no doctor so the babies died. When it looked as if it were going to happen again, I wanted to come to the hospital because I didn't want the same thing to happen, but it did. I was too late. All three have been stillborn.

It happens to other women in the village, too, because we don't have a health facility nearby. The only thing that would help is if we had health care near us. If a mother needed to deliver she could go to the nearest hospital before she suffered a long, difficult labor. So that is the only solution. But with no health facility, I think the same cases will happen again."

Dr. Shafiqa Kakar, Khost, Afghanistan

"Some patients come to MSF's hospital in Khost from far away and they cannot travel during the night due to security issues. Some patients have told us they were not able to come to the hospital when there was shooting and fighting, even though they were in labor or bleeding. Instead, they went to the nearby health centers. But some public health centers only have staff working in the morning. There are also private clinics that will induce the patients when they are not yet in labor, and sometimes the baby or the mother dies. Uterine rupture and obstructed labor are common. Many patients come to our hospital after having been induced in the private clinics. They come when they have complications, such as fetal distress. It happens a lot. The patients come to MSF because we have free medical care. In the public hospital if patients need a Caesarean section, they have to buy the medicines themselves from the bazaar, including the antibiotics needed after the C-section. Women also come because we only have female medical staff. Even if a woman is at risk of dying, she doesn't want to be examined by a man. Of course, there are not many female doctors in Khost. We have seven female doctors in the whole province. One of them is working with MSF."

Maternal Health Before And After Childbirth

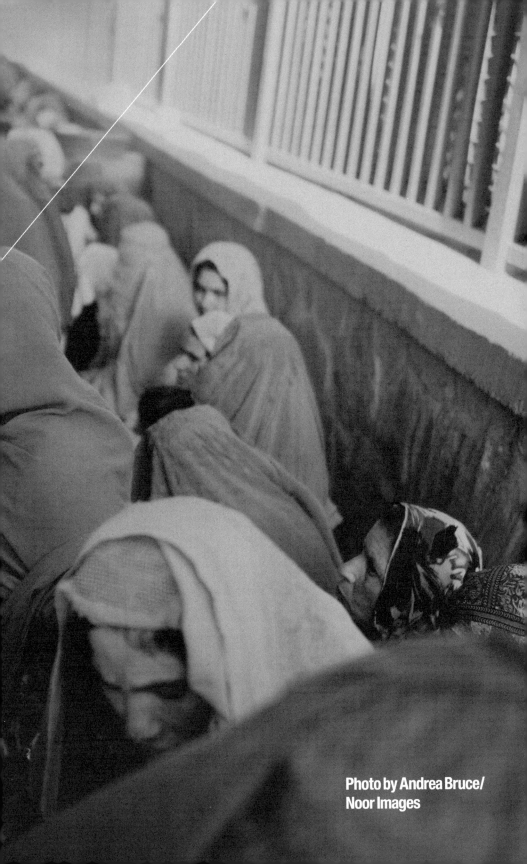

Photo by Andrea Bruce/
Noor Images

Chapter 2
Maternal Health Before and After Childbirth

The Lead-Up To Birth: Essential Antenatal Care
By Nele Segers, Midwife,
with Olivia Hill, RN, RM, BSc, MSc, and Eva Deplecker, Midwife

One morning in Gogrial, South Sudan, Grace arrived in our emergency room with her newborn baby. She was worried because he was sick and refusing to take her breast milk. When we examined the baby we found that he had tetanus, a disease both common and dangerous for newborns that is caused by exposure to a deadly bacterium.

Hundreds of thousands of babies die every year from neonatal tetanus, many in rural areas where it's very difficult to practice good hygiene. These babies might have been delivered by someone with dirty hands, or their umbilical cords might have been cut with a dirty razor or knife, or they might have been dressed with unclean material.

Tetanus has no cure, but it is preventable, and all women of childbearing age should receive vaccinations for the disease. This is a standard part of antenatal care (ANC). The vaccine protects the mother and her tetanus antibodies, once transferred to her baby, protect her child, too.

When we asked Grace if she had received her tetanus vaccination as part of her ANC, though, she replied that she had never had any ANC at all. The odds of her newborn surviving were not very good. Somewhere between 10 and 60 percent of babies with tetanus will survive as long as they get hospital care (the true survival rate is hard to quantify since so many babies die at home and their deaths go unreported, but we do know 100 percent of babies with tetanus will die if they do not get hospital care).

MSF offers reproductive health care in more than one-third of our projects, and ANC is part of the package. Many government health systems in developing countries offer the service as well. But in too many places, expectant mothers either cannot access it or do not fully take advantage of it. That was what happened in Grace's case, and now, because she had not gotten ANC and the tetanus vaccination offered as part of it, her baby's life was hanging in the balance.

We admitted Grace's boy and administered antibiotics, but he was not doing well. To nourish him, we ran a tube through his nose into his stomach. I explained to Grace and her husband that she and the baby needed to stay at the MSF hospital. The baby was running an extremely high fever and standard prodecures were not lowering it. As a last resort, we cooled the baby with ice. Under most circumstances, there's no way I would do this, but nothing else had been effective. Luckily, the ice worked. The baby's fever abated, and he gradually recovered from tetanus.

Later, the parents agreed to do a videotaped interview, something we could then use to convince other pregnant women to come in for at least two ANC visits before they delivered. We stressed the two visits because the tetanus vaccine must be given to an unimmunized woman in two doses, usually during the first and second ANC visits. I hoped that a local husband and wife speaking in their own language could better communicate why couples should come in for ANC when they were expecting a child.

Grace, her husband, her sister, and another family member all participated enthusiastically. Their experience had left them convinced about the need for ANC. At the end, her husband declared, "Next time I'll even force her to sit on the back of my bicycle while I take her the 35 kilometers to the center—twice!—so that she'll have the tetanus vaccine!"

When MSF opens a new project in an emergency, such as a conflict or natural disaster, we make the provision of obstetric care a priority. The team also provides basic ANC services to all pregnant women. This includes performing basic examinations, identifying potential complications, offering nutritional supplements, advising mothers on the benefits of delivering in a health facility, providing tetanus vaccinations and working to prevent or treat anemia and malaria—since malaria, which is endemic in many places MSF works, can cause pregnant women to give birth prematurely.

Once a team has established a baseline level of care, they will add more services as quickly as they can. The World Health Organization recommends that women have at least four ANC visits during each pregnancy, one visit in the first trimester of pregnancy, one in the second, and two more during the third. During the visits, a midwife should also test and treat the mother for anemia, malnutrition, sexually transmitted infections, HIV, and hypertension (high blood pressure)—whichever that apply.

Blood pressure is a key area of focus, since it can lead to pre-eclampsia and then eclampsia, a severe constellation of problems that can threaten the lives of the fetus and the mother. Along with obstructed labor, infections, severe bleeding and unsafe abortion, eclampsia is one of the five main causes of maternal mortality.

One reason ANC is such a crucial part of the effort to reduce maternal and newborn morbidity and mortality is that it connects women to the idea of delivering in a health facility. During ANC visits, midwives can talk with the mother about her birth plan. Where will she deliver? How will she get there? What transportation will she use? Will she have money for it? What happens if something goes wrong?

Ideally, as part of this conversation, midwives can convince women that their best and safest option would be to deliver at a hospital that has trained attendants and can handle serious complications, should they arise. But if the woman insists on delivering at home, the midwives then need to tell them how to recognize danger signs, so they know at what point they should be sure to seek out emergency care.

MSF staff carried out
712,278
antenatal consultations
at 131 projects in 2013.

In developed countries, many women make far more than four ANC visits, but they have options that people in places with limited to nonexistent health systems do not. The WHO reports that between 2006 and 2013 only 38 percent of pregnant women in low-income countries made at least four antenatal care visits.[i] That rate would be even lower in more isolated rural areas like Gogrial.

One reason for this is a sense that preventative care—going in for treatment before something is evidently wrong—is not part of customary health-seeking behavior in many places. Basic needs such as finding food or water or firewood seem far more pressing. What's more, if they do make the journey to a health facility, which by itself can take up half a day or more, they may have to spend hours at the facility, which might not seem worthwhile.

MSF tries to persuade more women to come for ANC by offering incentives such as mosquito nets or soap, which are important for their families' health. Where possible, MSF runs mobile clinics to outlying villages for ANC visits, bringing the care to the communities, but MSF teams can only cover limited areas. There are always women further afield who are beyond the teams' reach.

On average, MSF teams usually see women coming in for one or two ANC visits, usually late in their pregnancies. MSF has had to adapt to this reality, so staff work to provide the most possible benefit from every visit—since it may be the only time a woman gets any medical care before she delivers.

When women who have not received ANC come in to deliver, MSF health staff run easily administered tests for syphilis, gonorrhea, and HIV, and after birth, will offer counseling and treatment if any of the tests are positive.

The norm for women in many places where MSF works is homebirth, often with the assistance of a traditional birth attendant (TBA). TBAs are highly respected members of their communities who are upholding a tradition that stretches back generations. Those I've met have spent decades delivering babies after having apprenticed with their predecessors. They are frequently a pregnant woman's only connection to maternal care of any kind, and many women prefer the idea of giving birth at home with a TBA to the notion of going to a medical facility. For women with complications in birth, however, TBAs are not enough. They do not have the skills nor the medical materials to prevent women from dying.

Midwives talk about the "three delays"[ii] that can kill a mother in labor or her baby. The first stems from an assumption or hope that a TBA is all they need, so they do not seek out any other pre-delivery assistance, and then do not go to a properly resourced medical facility when complications arise. Few would-be mothers can recognize these complications by themselves, and the TBA might not know how to either. But if they don't know how to see that the placenta is in the wrong place, for instance, they're likely to wait too long before heading to the hospital.

To address this, MSF tries to build relationships with TBAs, so they know what services we offer. We also provide trainings for them on recognizing potential complications. We do not train TBAs to do home deliveries, but MSF sometimes hires them to provide other assistance in our maternity wards. The goal is the same: we want them to bring mothers to our hospitals or to other facilities where they can receive the skilled birth attendance that can mean the difference between life and death.

Working with TBAs can be controversial, because many people see them as an obstacle preventing women from getting proper care. Some countries, like Uganda and Sierra Leone, have gone so far as to ban TBAs from practicing at all. Nigeria began regulating the practice of traditional medicine, including TBAs, in the 1970s and started creating model traditional health care clinics with registered care providers.[iii] But the fact remains that in many places TBAs are the only option women have, particularly women living in rural areas, far from the resources and hospitals of bigger cities. In Masisi, Democratic Republic of Congo, our ANC team would walk through the bush for hours, three times a week to reach villages that would otherwise have no access to maternal care. The TBAs are often our first point of contact and in many cases they are helpful. But we're also aware that we're asking them to send people to us, which means forgoing income they would have made.

The second delay is when a woman cannot reach a place with skilled medical care. It might be too far away. Or there might not be any transportation available, or the roads are too dangerous, or a husband or parent doesn't think it's worth spending the amount of money it requires. If a plan has already been worked out during the ANC process, it can pre-empt some of these factors.

The third delay is an absence of good quality care at a health facility. A mother could arrive at night when no skilled staff would be present. There may be staff but no drugs or equipment. In some places where medical care is supposedly free, facilities lack medical materials or even medicines, and the woman has to provide her own. If she can't provide these often expensive items, she may be ignored, mistreated, or denied admission.

MSF and other health care providers have implemented strategies to address the three delays. The most notable one involves bringing women closer to care by offering them the chance to spend their last weeks of pregnancy living in safe, comfortable maternity waiting houses. These have been extremely successful—and some women are even referred by TBAs with whom we've established relationships. In Masisi, the mobile ANC team identifies women who are likely to need emergency care—those with previous Caesarean sections, pre-eclampsia, or several previous births. Nearer to the woman's birth date, the TBA in her community walks with her to the waiting home, which is located on the grounds of MSF's hospital. Women receive free food, a bed, and the space to rest in the company of other pregnant women. When it is time to deliver, they do not have far to go to receive skilled care and, if needed, surgical care. The waiting house can receive more than 70 women at a time and it has been in high demand since it opened in 2009.

The MSF team in Aroressa, Ethiopia, saw the same high demand when they opened a maternity waiting home in the isolated, mountainous area where they were working. One woman, Fayza, was near the end of her pregnancy when she was referred by our outreach team to our maternity waiting home. If she had stayed in the mountains where she lived until delivery, the local clinic staff, which lacked trained midwives, may have sent her to the understaffed, undersupplied health center nearby. They could not have brought her by car to our health center. The roads were so bad that we had to use horses, and even they had trouble in the mountains.

Because Fayza reached us early enough and stayed in our maternity waiting home, she could give birth in our clinic. In her second stage of labor, her baby's heartbeat began to sound very faint. We determined that the baby was in fetal distress, but we had the necessary equipment and we delivered him alive. Again, if Fayza had delivered in the mountains, her baby could have died or suffered brain damage from a lack of oxygen during labor. The maternity waiting home—and her decision to stay in it—almost certainly saved her baby's life.

We had started with just a few rooms because we did not know whether mothers would respond to a maternity waiting home in Aroressa; it can be hard to predict what will be acceptable in a given community. Whereas in Masisi mothers are admitted to the waiting home if they face a high risk of complications, in Ethiopia I had to weigh both the risk of complications and the distance the mother lived from the clinic, because transportation was such a major issue. Still, within one week of establishing this service, we had 20 patients. We quickly grew from a few rooms to a large tent to an entire house. Maternity waiting homes can be costly to operate, but given the impact, and the lives saved, we were convinced that it was more than worthwhile.

In some regions, particular issues must be addressed: one is female genital mutilation (FGM). There are places where MSF works in which the practice is common and nearly all the pregnant mothers a midwife sees will have undergone some type of FGM.

Usually performed on a girl when she is very young, FGM can lead to many harmful complications in the course of a woman's life. It is most often during deliveries, however, that MSF deals with problems related to FGM. About 15 percent of all women with FGM have undergone infibulation,[iv] in which the circumciser narrows a girl's vaginal opening by cutting and repositioning part of the labia to create a seal. When the girl's legs are tied together for a period of time the seal fuses.

A woman who has been infibulated may have to be de-infibulated to give birth. If this is performed by an unskilled person in an unclean environment, the de-infibulation can cause obstetric complications that affect mother and baby. Obstructed labor can lead to hemorrhaging in the mother and a lack of oxygen for the baby, which can leave both mother and child traumatized and vulnerable to infection. To avoid such dangers, women with FGM need to be encouraged to deliver in a health facility.

It used to be that ANC was designed to help health workers identify which women were at risk according to certain criteria, and then to decide who needed to deliver in a hospital based on that criteria. However, maternal mortality did not consequently decline, because complications very often cannot be predicted. Many, but not all, problems are preventable with good care, so MSF's goal is to have all women come to the hospital to deliver—even if they only make one or two ANC visits during their pregnancy.

MSF has adapted its approach to antenatal care to the realities of women's lives and the competing needs they face in the places where we work. There are some limitations to this approach, some inherent frustrations as well. But there is still much we can do and accomplish. We can establish maternity waiting homes and make sure women in the area know about them. We can connect and form relationships with TBAs. We can give women incentives to come to ANC, we can run mobile medical units, and we can provide testing and counseling during labor. And we do all these things in an effort to ensure that women have the greatest possible access to emergency obstetric care. Insofar as ANC can connect women with these services, it can help save their lives.

The Risk Doesn't End When the Baby Is Born: The Importance of Postnatal Care
By Debbie Price, CNM, DrPH

A few years ago, I was in central Chad, working in a field hospital that our team had established inside a camp for around 170,000 internally displaced people. I was doing ward rounds in the maternity unit, a standard practice in hospitals where the midwife goes from bed to bed, examining mothers and their babies, making note of who should be seen by the doctor, who needed tests or treatments, who could use extra support with breastfeeding, and who could be discharged that day. Suddenly, a woman ran into the ward and told us that her neighbor, a woman named Mariyamu, was badly ill. Some team members and I followed her to the neighbor's hut, where we found Mariyamu lying on a thin mattress, moaning, with her newborn baby lying next to her. Mariyamu was 17. Days earlier, she had given birth to the baby, her first, inside the hut with the assistance of a traditional birth attendant. Mariyamu's few belongings—a cooking pot, a jerry can, some plastic plates and cups—were arranged neatly around them, but the young woman was clearly in a state of distress.

We checked the baby, who seemed fine. When I examined Mariyamu, I saw that she was feverish, her lower abdomen was tender, and she was enveloped in a foul odor, which indicated a postnatal infection. Puerperal infection, which is sometimes called "childbed fever," describes any bacterial infection of the genital tract that occurs after childbirth. Most commonly caused by the person assisting in the delivery's failure to wash their hands or otherwise practice good hygiene, it affects about 4.5 percent of all birth mothers, which amounts to roughly six million cases per year.[v] Another contributing factor is retained tissue—fragments of placenta or bits of membranes from the amniotic sac that did not come out during delivery.

Untreated infections, including puerperal sepsis, account for 15 percent of all maternal deaths.[vi] But when a woman is assisted during delivery by a skilled birth attendant, the risk of infection is reduced by half. A trained midwife knows to make sure anything that touches the baby is clean. When the placenta is delivered, the midwife sees that all the membranes are carefully teased out, and she will check the delivered placenta to make sure it is not missing any fragments. Only 46 percent of births in developing countries, however, are assisted by skilled attendants.[vii]

We took Mariyamu to our postnatal ward and removed the retained tissue from her uterus. We then started her on antibiotics for her infection and other medication to ease her pain. We examined her baby, Rosalie, more closely, and she was still fine. Mother and child stayed at the hospital for five days, during which time Mariyamu recovered and we helped her establish breastfeeding. When she was healthy, she returned home with Rosalie.

The first six weeks following childbirth, the postnatal period, is the most dangerous time for mother and baby. Seventy-five percent of all neonatal deaths occur in the first week of the postnatal period.[viii] More than 35 percent of maternal deaths occur during this time, too; most, in fact, happen within the first 24 hours.[ix] The main causes are excessive blood loss/hemorrhage and pregnancy-related high blood pressure (including eclampsia). Those who die in the second to fourth weeks most often succumb to infection. Mariyamu would have been one of those women had she not received help.

One of the major differences between giving birth in developed and undeveloped countries is access to postnatal care (PNC). It stands in contrast to access to antenatal care (ANC), which has been recognized for decades as an important part of maternity care and is often the only component of it that a woman ever receives. Whereas ANC has benefitted from longstanding campaigns in developing countries by the World Health Organization, ministries of health, and non-governmental organizations, the importance of PNC has gotten much less recognition. In 2013, MSF staff conducted roughly one-third, as many PNC consultations as ANC consultations.

Over the past few decades, as more and better data have been captured, the medical community has realized that for many pregnant women, life-threatening complications cannot be identified during ANC. They have also seen that many maternal deaths occur in the postnatal period, underscoring the importance of PNC. It was asserted in a 1996 study published in *International Journal of Gynecology & Obstetrics* that if PNC were provided with the same dedication as ANC in developing countries, around 90 percent of maternal deaths that occur during the month after delivery could be avoided.[x]

MSF staff try to see women twice for postnatal care. The first visit should happen within the first week of the baby's life if delivery occurred at a medical facility. If the mother gave birth at home, she and the child should ideally be examined within 24 hours. In either case, a midwife or a specially trained nurse checks for danger signs that would indicate medical issues that require immediate attention for the mother. These would include heavy vaginal bleeding, fevers, severe headaches, or hypertension. At the same time, the midwife checks the baby to see if he or she is breathing and eating well and if there are any signs of jaundice or problems with eyes or umbilicus.

Babies usually get vitamin K during the first visit to help their blood clot. They also get tetracycline eye ointment to protect them from neonatal conjunctivitis, which can cause blindness. Babies should also receive a "birth dose" of vaccinations to prevent tuberculosis, polio, and hepatitis B before they begin routine vaccinations at six weeks old. If the mother did not receive a tetanus vaccine during ANC, the midwife or nurse will administer it during the first PNC visit, along with vitamin A and ferrous sulfate/folic acid supplements. They'll talk with the mother about healthy birth spacing, and if she wants contraception, they will provide it. MSF will also give undernourished mothers supplemental food and HIV-positive mothers antitretroviral treatment, if they are not already receiving it. The staff will also ensure that a baby born to a mother with HIV who is not in a program to prevent transmission gets preventive treatment for HIV. [See Chapter 6: PMTCT]

The second visit should come at about six weeks, when the baby starts receiving routine vaccinations. Tying PNC to vaccinations gives women an incentive to receive the care, as most mothers know the value of vaccines and they seem to appreciate receiving both services in one visit. Mothers will have learned about postnatal hygiene, nutrition, and sex, as well as breastfeeding, how to care for the baby, and how to identify potential danger signs in the first visit and these things will be covered again in the second.

Another general benefit of receiving PNC is that the mother and baby may be spared harmful traditional practices. They'll be warned not to give the baby anything made with water that's not clean—weak tea, rice water, or diluted animal milk, for instance—which can lead to diarrhea. They should also not allow any unclean substances, such as animal dung or ash, to come into contact with the baby's umbilical cord at the time of birth.

The benefits PNC brings in the hours and weeks after birth are numerous, but the challenge is persuading women to come for the care. The same measures that MSF health workers employ to draw women to ANC can also work for PNC: they offer basic items like a towel and soap as incentives, and make sure to have extra staff on hand in our projects on market day, when most women are out in the biggest population center in the area and therefore more likely to come in.

These days, I work as a specialist advisor on sexual and reproductive health for MSF. Among other duties, I visit projects around the world to help teams improve their services. In 2011, for example, I went to both Pakistan and Bangladesh, where I spent time with two maternity teams that were trying to solve the question of how to get PNC to women in their catchment area. Each came up with a unique solution.

In Kuchlak, an Afghan refugee community in Pakistan's Balochistan Province, the staff were encouraging women to stay in the birthing unit for at least four hours after delivery so they and newborns could receive preventive care and be monitored for any postnatal issues. This worked well with some women who lived close by the clinic, but many of the patients came from as far as 90 miles (150 km) away. They were the women and the newborns the team was most worried about. They would often arrive in a hired vehicle that waited outside while the mother gave birth, and would leave immediately after. It was highly unlikely that they'd be able to get any PNC in their communities and equally unlikely that they would later make the long journey back to the MSF clinic for follow-up care.

Most women, whether they lived nearby or far away, needed a male attendant in order to leave the house; usually it was their husbands. This was a problem for couples living far away because the man would have to miss a day's work if his wife stayed at the clinic for treatment and evaluation.

Our staff would hear stories about these patients when a neighbor or relative would come in to get health care and mention what had befallen a new mother in their community. Most of the stories we heard had bad outcomes, and while they could not be considered a scientific measure of what happens to women who do not receive PNC, they were nonetheless important indicators.

To address some of these issues, the team in Kuchlak started providing PNC home visits, when and where possible. A Lady Health Visitor (LHV, a professional position similar to a midwife) would come to a woman's home during the first and second weeks after delivery. In each visit, the LHV would spend at least 15 minutes with the mother, providing her and her baby with standard PNC and any other treatment that was necessary. The LHV was accompanied by female health educator, who gathered the women in the household and talked to them about vaccinations, breastfeeding, hygiene and other important information. A male health educator spoke to the men of the community about various relevant health issues as well.

This approach proved successful. The LHVs were soon seeing up to 150 women per month. This was in a very volatile region, however, and due to insecurity, the team had to curtail the home visits. They became another casualty of conflict.

MSF has implemented home visits by skilled professionals in other contexts as well, but it's often not sustainable because sending out staff by vehicle can get prohibitively expensive. A better long-term solution has been training local community health workers to check for danger signs in mothers and babies while also conducting health education sessions. When needed, they can refer patients who need treatment to MSF facilities.

In 2013, MSF staff provided 117,150 postnatal consultations in 116 projects. This is about one-third of the number of patients who came for ANC. Nevertheless, the numbers have been slowly increasing over the years.

If a clinic or hospital already offers ANC, very little additional work and expense is required to add PNC. The staff needs are the same, and only a little additional training is necessary. But staff focused on PNC will often encounter the same difficulties faced by those trying to provide ANC. Women often have competing needs, and the more immediate issues take precedence. They may live far from the nearest clinic or hospital and lack money for transport. The roads may be dangerous. They may not be used to seeking preventative care.

The greatest challenge, though, is the lack of awareness about PNC and its benefits. This was starkly evident when I visited the Kutupalong camp in Bangladesh. Kutupalong was an unofficial settlement inhabited by members of the long-ostracized Rohingya ethnic group who had migrated from Myanmar. They were not given any state services and thus had no access to health care. MSF began providing primary medical care on the camp's outskirts and eventually established a maternity center that offered emergency obstetric care services, ANC and PNC.

When I visited, I was told that many women came in for the ANC component of the reproductive health program but virtually no one was coming for post-partum care. A retrospective study in the camp showed a high incidence of newborn deaths within the first few days of life. The team was making an effort to communicate the importance of PNC in the crucial days after delivery, but there were a host of obstacles that needed to be overcome.

In Rohingya communities, women often observe a lying-in period of up to six weeks, during which mothers and their babies do not leave the home or do any housework or fieldwork. Naturally, if a woman cannot leave her home, she cannot come in for PNC. Our staff went to the camp's elders, who are called *majees*, and explained that the lack of PNC was a primary reason so many newborns were dying. The *majees* listened and resolved the problem by proclaiming that the MSF clinic could be considered an extension of the women's homes.

Now, thanks to clear communication, coming to PNC was acceptable. The team just had to figure out how to get new mothers to the clinic.

As a matter of protocol, MSF provides vitamin K and preventive eye treatment to newborns—ideally in the first two days of life, but the medications are effective up to seven days after delivery. The team connected this to their messaging about PNC, casting both as critical aspects of mother and child health that could be provided in the days after a baby was born.

Quickly, we saw that mothers who hadn't been coming in earlier were now arriving at our clinic seeking both the medications for their newborns and general PNC services. Virtually every new mother in the camp came in for at least one PNC visit within the first few months of the campaign. The numbers later fell and then leveled off at around 40 percent of new mothers—not what it was during the best days, but far better than it was before we started the campaign, and better than the average at most MSF projects.

While PNC is typically overshadowed by other aspects of maternal care, MSF has increasingly made it an extension of the effort to convince women to seek out skilled assistance during deliveries. More women still seem to respond to offers of ANC, however, as if they believe that once a child is born, there is much less to worry about—even in places where childhood mortality remains a pressing issue. According to the WHO, for instance, PNC programs in sub-Saharan Africa are among the least utilized of all reproductive and child health programs.[xi]

MSF's PNC strategy has three main points. First, PNC services need to be promoted during the comparatively well-attended ANC sessions. ANC, skilled delivery, PNC, and newborn care should be presented as one essential program of care.

Second, the message about PNC must also be spread throughout communities. The idea of preventive care should be explained; even if mother and baby are healthy and have no problems, they can still benefit from the service. People in the community also must be made aware of dangers to watch for in mothers and babies.

And third, until all women have access to skilled delivery, MSF staff must establish relationships with traditional birth attendants to improve their referral of women for post-partum care.

With more than 36 percent of maternal deaths occurring during the postnatal period, it's clear how important PNC is and the impact it can have. It is relatively easy to provide and it gets results. MSF's data for all projects that offer the service show that in 2013, staff detected illnesses in 11 percent of mothers and 14 percent of babies who were seen for postnatal care. They diagnosed 5,571 women with puerperal sepsis, wound infection, post-partum depression and other illnesses, and 5,420 babies, many with early-onset neonatal sepsis from bad hygienic practices during home deliveries. All were treated and their lives were saved.

This is why MSF sees PNC as a vital service for women and their children, and why we think it is so important to have it be part of the continuum of care—ANC, skilled delivery, PNC and newborn care—that health systems and organizations aspire to provide.

[i] WHO, Global Health Observatory. "Antenatal Care." Accessed December 2014. http://www.who.int/gho/maternal_health/reproductive_health/antenatal_care_text/en/

[ii] Sereen Thaddeus and Deborah Maine, "Too Far to Walk: Maternal Mortality in Context." Social Science Medicine, Vol. 38. No. 8, pp. 1091-1110, 1994. http://www.researchgate.net/publication/46505614_Too_far_to_walk_Maternal_mortality_in_context/links/00b495283bb-7b3ece3000000

[iii] WHO, Essential Medicines and Health Products portal. "Legal Status of Traditional Medicine and Complementary/Alternative Medicine: A Worldwide Review." 2001. p. 29-30. Accessed December 2014. http://apps.who.int/medicinedocs/pdf/h2943e/h2943e.pdf

[iv] Frances A. Althaus, "Female Circumcision: Rite of Passage Or Violation of Rights?" Guttmacher Institute. International Family Planning Perspectives. Vol. 23, No. 3, September 1997. http://www.guttmacher.org/pubs/journals/2313097.html

[v] Carla AbouZahr, "Global burden of maternal death and disability," British Medical Bulletin. 2003; 67: p. 7. http://bmb.oxfordjournals.org/content/67/1/1.full.pdf

[vi] Nawal M. Nour, "An Introduction to Maternal Mortality," Review of Obstetric Gynecology, Spring 2008; 1(2): p. 77–81. http://www.ncbi.nlm.nih.gov/pmc/articles/PMC2505173/

[vii] WHO, Global Health Observatory. Situation and Trends. "Skilled attendants at birth." Accessed December 2014. http://www.who.int/gho/maternal_health/skilled_care/skilled_birth_attendance_text/en/

[viii] UNICEF, "Maternal and Newborn Health." 2012. http://www.unicef.org/health/index_maternalhealth.html

[ix] Kassebaum et al, "Global, regional, and national levels and causes of maternal mortality during 1990-2013: a systematic analysis for the Global Burden of Disease study 2013." The Lancet. Vol. 384 No. 9947.pp 980-1004. http://download.thelancet.com/pdfs/journals/lancet/PIIS0140673614606966.pdf?id=eaaMohvADxp3pdj6-IWOu

[x] X.F. Li, J.A. Fortney, M. Kotelchuck, L.H. Glover, "The postpartum period: the key to maternal mortality." International Journal of Gynaecology and Obstetrics 1996;54:1-10.

[xi] WHO, The Partnership for Maternal, Newborn & Child Health. "Opportunities for Africa's Newborns: Practical data, policy, and programmatic support for newborn care in Africa." 2006. p. 79. http://www.who.int/pmnch/media/publications/oanfullreport.pdf

STORIES FROM PATIENTS

Shalila, 24, Khost, Afghanistan

"I am having some contractions now. I want more contractions. I asked the midwife here to give me an injection for more contractions, but she said MSF would not give this to me. I want to end this problem. I have leg pain. [The pregnancy] is too heavy for me. [*Patients in labor in Afghanistan and Pakistan frequently ask for injections of Oxytocin in order to deliver faster. The drug is safe if it is administered to a patient with a medical need for it through infusion, with the dosage gradually increased. However, misused injections of oxytocin are dangerous. They can cause uterine rupture and the baby can die.*]

When I delivered in private clinics previously, they gave me injections to induce the contractions, but MSF doctors told me the injection is not good for my health. Now I know and I don't go to private clinics for an injection.

I have done two antenatal checkups for this pregnancy. My tummy was too big so I went for antenatal care. I didn't know it was twins. If my stomach was not this big, I would not have gone for a checkup. In my village, women usually don't go for antenatal care.

The road here was okay, but I will not travel after 8 p.m. There are robbers and they stop the cars and steal money. Even if we need to go to the hospital during the night, we will not go; we will wait until at least 5 a.m. to travel.

Sometimes the road is blocked because of the fighting between the armed forces and opposition groups. It usually happens during the night. We hear shootings sometimes, and we will stay at home if there is shooting."

Asunta, 20, Aweil, South Sudan

"When people in our village are sick we go to a private clinic and things are expensive. Drugs are expensive. Consultations are expensive.

I came here to the hospital because of labor pain. I have had the pain for two days. My parents called the traditional birth attendant to come and attend the delivery. The birth attendant stayed with me until the morning. I went to the church to pray, then, after morning prayers, I took public transport to the hospital. We don't have maternal care in the village.

When I arrived here, the midwife confirmed that I was in labor, and I delivered.

Whenever I want to come to the hospital it is easy for me to use public transport. I've come here for antenatal care during previous pregnancies. I'm not like other mothers because our area is a little bit close to the town.

The best way to help the mothers is to send a health educator into the villages to tell them to come to the hospital when they fall sick. It is very important."

Odette, 23, Kabezi, Burundi

"I gave birth to my third child yesterday—a girl—by Caesarean section. It was my first C-section: my other two children were born naturally at the Kabezi district hospital.

As I was reaching my due date, I was really scared. I could feel that this pregnancy was different from the others. With the previous two I felt as if my belly was dropping lower as I approached the birth. But for this one, it didn't—I actually felt as if the baby was moving up into my chest. Also, instead of feeling contractions, I just had terrible pains in my abdomen.

At home, people were trying to reassure me that the pregnancy just hadn't reached term yet. They said that I should wait, that things would happen naturally. But I really felt things that were not like my previous pregnancies. And as I'm not used to giving birth at home, I thought it would be better to come here, where there would be people on hand who could help me.

About a week ago, I went to the district hospital to get a consultation as per normal. They told me that I should come here to the MSF hospital. But when I arrived here the staff told me that my pregnancy hadn't reached term, and that I had to wait a bit. I really didn't feel well so I said instead of going home I'd prefer to stay here with the other women in the maternity waiting home. A week passed, and yesterday I gave birth by Caesarean section. *[Odette's labor was obstructed.]*

I am feeling a lot better than I did yesterday. Save for the pain of the wound I have from the operation, I feel good. I'll stay here as long as it takes to get back on my feet then go home."

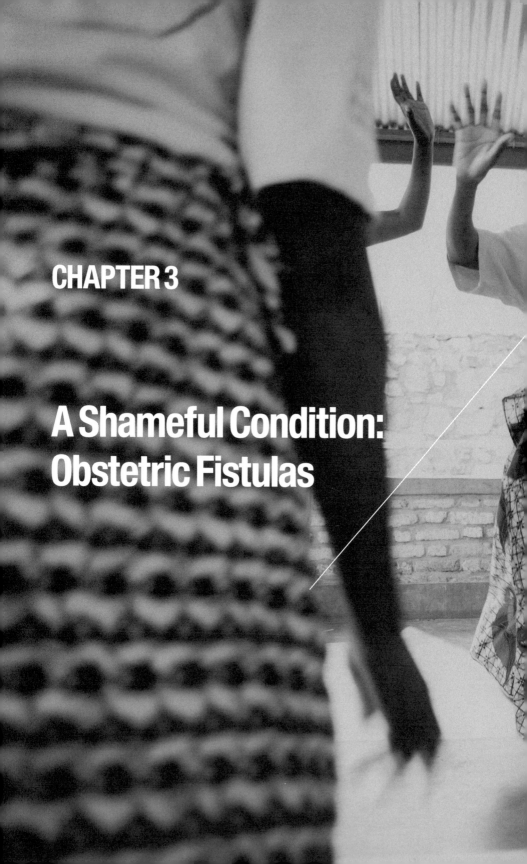

CHAPTER 3

A Shameful Condition: Obstetric Fistulas

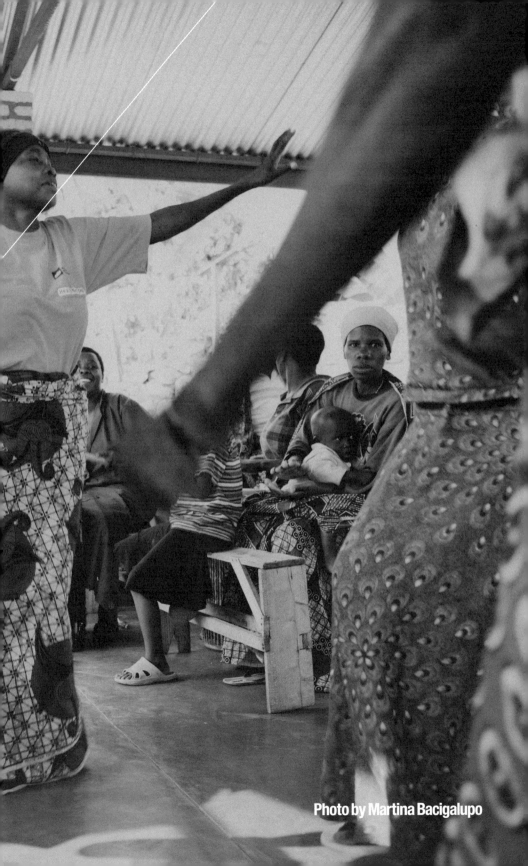

Photo by Martina Bacigalupo

Chapter 3
A Shameful Condition: Obstetric Fistulas

Contributions from Michiel Lekkerkerker, MD

Dhaayo and Haldhaa, both 17, were admitted to the first fistula camp MSF organized, in Galkayo South, Somalia, in November 2007.

They had become pregnant at 14, and when it came time to deliver, they went through days of excruciating labor at home. In the end, their babies arrived stillborn. In one way, they were fortunate: they survived while most girls and women who experience prolonged obstructed labor with no skilled assistance will die due to uterine rupture. If the mother continues to have contractions while the baby's head is unable to descend into the birth canal, the womb can tear and the baby will be expelled into the abdominal cavity. The mother dies of blood loss from the torn uterus, and the baby dies as well.

This did not happen to Dhaayo and Haldhaa. They lived. But they soon noticed that they were no longer able to control their bladders, that they were "leaking" urine and feces involuntarily. The price they had paid for survival was an obstetric fistula.

An obstetric fistula is an opening between the vagina and the bladder that occurs during prolonged obstructed labor. As the hours pass and labor continues, the baby's skull presses the connective tissue between the vagina and the bladder against the pelvic bones. If this goes on for a while, the tissue can die and a hole can develop between the vagina and the bladder—a vesico-vaginal fistula. It can also happen to tissue between the vagina and the rectum, causing a recto-vaginal fistula. When this happens the woman will lose stool through her vagina.

According to the best available data, 50,000 to 100,000 women develop fistulas every year, and at least two million women and girls are suffering from fistulas at any given time.[i] (It's widely believed that these numbers are significantly lower than the reality.) Most women develop fistulas young, many in their teens.[ii] And while not immediately life-threatening, fistulas bring profound consequences.

Women living with a fistula are frequently relegated to life as an outcast. A husband will turn his wife out of the house, parents will refuse to help her, and co-wives or neighbors will ridicule and ostracize her. In places where a woman's life is entirely dependent on being part of a family, expulsion can make survival extraordinarily difficult. If she doesn't find help, she will bear this burden for the rest of her life, and help in many places is unavailable.

In 2007, MSF began running "fistula camps" to provide specialized fistula repair surgery in places where the needs were most evident. The camps last around six weeks. The first phase involves getting out the word in the communities, letting people—especially women with fistulas—know they are happening and what they involve. An advance team then sets up tents with 40 to 80 beds near a functioning hospital and hires additional staff to assist.

Once the preparations have been made, a fistula surgeon arrives and spends the next month or so operating on several women each day. Once recovered, these women are led through exercises designed to help them regain control over muscles that had been rendered all but useless by the fistula.

In Galkayo, a remote, undeveloped part of a long-troubled country, we had worked with community health educators and medical staff at small health centers to spread a very basic message: "if you leak urine, you can be cured; come to the MSF fistula camp." We made announcements on radio stations as well, to get the word out even more widely. In all cases, we said that women must bring a caretaker, that they would have to follow the strict instructions given during the camp, and that success was not 100 percent guaranteed.

When we opened the door, 25 women with fistulas showed up. They sat silently on their beds, their heads and faces covered by their niqabs and veils in the stifling heat. They were hesitant, uncertain, likely worn down and possibly depressed by their experience of living with a fistula.

A few weeks later, most of the women had been operated on and had started recovery. I vividly remember the dramatic change in atmosphere. These women were now laughing, making jokes, encouraging each other. They were exhilarated. Fistula surgery meant having a second chance at life.

It's something I've seen many times since. In 2008, MSF organized a fistula camp in Dubié, South Kivu Province, in Democratic Republic of Congo (DRC). Among those who came were Michèle, 16, and Josine, 19. They had similar stories: early pregnancy, three days of obstructed labor at home, far from the closest available medical facilities. Their babies had died and they had both developed fistulas. Soon after, their husbands spurned them.

Deeply ashamed, Michèle returned to the home of her parents, who reluctantly took her back in, while Josine did likewise and gradually withdrew from the life she had led. "I used to work in the fields and I had friends," she told me. "But as soon as I realized that I had a fistula, I distanced myself from my community out of shame—because of being wet all the time and the smell I was spreading."

In all likelihood, Michèle, Josine, Dhaayo and Haldhaa experienced obstructed labor—and then fistulas—because they were young and their pelvises were too small for their children to pass through. It's often said that fistulas can result from early pregnancy or early marriage, but it's not that simple.

In the U.S., for instance, 305,420 babies were born to girls and young women 15 to 19 years old in 2012[iii] but there have been very few fistulas for a long time.[iv] Early pregnancy is a cause for concern everywhere around the world, but fistulas occur in developing countries because of the lack of access to emergency obstetric care. Even where fistula repair surgery is available, there needs to be more fistula prevention, which is to say more access to emergency care, to skilled birth attendants, and to properly outfitted medical facilities.

That remains MSF's top priority when it comes to the health of pregnant and delivering girls and young women. Fistula repair projects can achieve wonderful things, but they should always complement obstetric care programs, not serve as a stand-in for them.

Fistulas continue to be a hidden problem, relegated to the shadows, affecting women in societies that see them as subordinate and where those who endure them are stigmatized and shrouded in shame.
The price of silence is high, even if some of the affects are not immediately evident. Women with fistulas frequently drink as little as possible in order to leak as little urine as they can, but as the urine becomes more concentrated, it smells stronger. What's more, not drinking can lead to chronic bladder, kidney and skin infections, and bladder stones. And over time, the vagina may become shorter, narrower and less flex-

ible, hampering a woman's ability to have sex and lessening the possibility of surgical repair.

Women with a fistula often end up in a downward spiral. Many can support themselves only as sex workers and are continuously exposed to sexually transmitted infections, including HIV, which heightens their vulnerability and lessens their chances of being cured.

If a woman already has children, or gets the fistula when she's older, or has the support of the people around her, she may have a better chance of remaining connected to her community. But the best protection against the consequences of having a fistula is early repair. In the best case, that would be within months of its occurrence.

During a visit to the fistula repair department at Mohammed Murtala Hospital in Kano, Nigeria, in 2006, I met 35-year-old Azalee. She had been living with a fistula for 12 years. Unable to find a job, she'd been forced to earn her living as a sex worker. She was now suffering from all the complications mentioned above. I still remember how devastated she was when she was told that it was too late for her to be repaired.

There are fistula repair centers in larger African cities like Kano and Katsina in Nigeria, Bamako in Mali, and Addis Ababa in Ethiopia. Some are well-known. However, doctors trained in doing fistula repairs in these countries tend to be concentrated in capital cities, along with relatively accessible obstetric facilities. Their services remain out of reach for women in rural areas.

When sexual and reproductive health became a priority for MSF in the late 1990s, and its antenatal and obstetric services were expanding—particularly in conflict-ridden places like Sierra Leone, Liberia, DRC, South Sudan, and Somalia—fistulas gradually emerged as a serious reproductive health problem. We could see that a great need was being covered only marginally, often with poor quality care, so I worked with Dr. Kees Waaldijk, the world's most experienced fistula surgeon, to organize a training program for MSF gynecologists and surgeons.

Dr. Waaldijk, a Dutchman, has been doing fistula repair surgeries in Nigeria for more than 25 years. With his help we established a small pool of MSF doctors who were well-trained in fistula repair, which we augmented by hiring specially trained surgeons from a Geneva-based association of Swiss urologists.

In 2007, when MSF began providing fistula care, teams carried out 195 operations. By 2011, the number had risen to 1,036, or almost seven percent of the repairs reported worldwide. In 2013, MSF provided 1,032 fistula repair surgeries. It's been heartening to be able to help more women, but we're always mindful of the fact that this is only a fraction of the new cases that develop each year.

Fistula care is much more than just mending the hole. It requires raising awareness, prevention, surgery, a caring attitude from the staff, and the patient's involvement.

There are only a few places in the world where high-quality fistula repair training is provided and space in these programs is limited. For MSF, it is not a one-off training; staff alternate between time spent training and time in the field. Most MSF doctors trained in fistula surgery have returned to Nigeria three or four times to complete their training with Dr. Waaldijk. Now they can be considered trainers themselves; they can continue to use their skills to assist women in need while also preparing others to do the same.

It's been difficult to train surgeons in the countries where MSF runs programs, however. Potential candidates might have other interests or they might have been assigned to other programs by their ministries of health. And fistula surgery is not easy. A lot of tissue loss can occur as a consequence of obstetric trauma, leaving less material to work with. Most fistulas are operated on through the vagina. Therefore, the handling of instruments can be difficult, because the operation field is limited and deep at the same time. An unsuccessful attempt to repair can result in additional scarring of the tissue, making things worse for the patient. The tissue can lose elasticity and become less usable for closure or reconstruction when another repair is attempted.

What's more, success over the long term is only likely if the patient is actively involved in her healing. Fistula pre- and postoperative care is not complex but patients must faithfully adhere to a few basic instructions: drink four to six liters of fluids per day, remain mobile at all times and do the exercises they learn, leave the urinary catheters in place, and avoid sex for four to six months after the operation. (Fistula patients are advised not to get pregnant within a year after repair, and advised that any future deliveries should be by Caesarean section.)

Preferably, staff on the fistula ward have professional nursing or midwifery diplomas, but it is equally important that they are caring, pragmatic, and disciplined. They must be able to motivate patients to take part in their own healing.

The change in atmosphere at our first fistula camp in South Galkayo resulted partly from the women's great relief at seeing an end to their suffering. But it was also an indication of how motivated the staff were. They created an atmosphere that made the patients see they were not alone, encouraging them to bond with their peers, bolstering their confidence, helping them find the courage to heal and then re-enter the society that had shunned them.

At a fistula program in Mali, I worked with a woman named Zeynabou. She was petite but too loud, too cheerful, and too radiant to be overlooked. I might have guessed she was about 45, but she was only 28.

She'd been a patient before she was a colleague. Pregnant at 13, she delivered a stillborn child after a lengthy, difficult labor and developed a fistula that went unattended for several years. Six more pregnancies all ended the same way, and she became an outcast in her community, miserable, isolated, unsure of her future.

Then she visited an MSF fistula camp, where her fistula was successfully repaired. Her life changed almost immediately, and she became the buoyant, confident, optimistic woman she is today. Wisely, MSF asked her to become the outreach ambassador for its fistula program, a post reserved for a former patient who is well-suited to the task of raising awareness about fistula prevention and repair.

In addition, she serves as the *maman village*, or hostess, of the fistula compound. She greets newly admitted patients and walks them through the routines of the camp, putting them at ease, encouraging them, and communicating to them why it's so important that they comply with the instructions they're given.

She performed her roles very well, serving as an excellent example to the new patients—a living illustration of what was possible for them. When I had to leave the project, she told me almost everything was fine again in her life except she didn't have children and a husband yet, so she proposed to me!

In some places, MSF runs one or two fistula camps per year. In others, it offers repair surgery as part of regular medical services. Both approaches use a well-established secondary-level obstetric facility as a point of departure—an acknowledgement that fistulas, as well as uterine rupture, are consequences of shortcomings with regard to emergency obstetric care.

The approach we take is chosen based on the circumstances: a camp may be the better choice if fistula surgeons are only available for a limited amount of time, if relatively few patients come because of insecurity and conflict, or because of particularly strong social stigma.

Working in a conflict zone may require projects to produce smaller footprints as well. I remember being in Somalia in 2007 when we had to quickly dismantle a fistula camp in Marere and move it—including patients, tents, water tanks, surgical equipment and staff—to Kismayo.

Another major challenge is patient follow-up, which is crucial because repaired fistulas take time to fully heal. The restored anatomy is fragile; a fresh fistula repair can easily break down during the first months after surgery, especially if sexual activity is resumed too soon.

There are two common reasons why patients don't appear for follow-up appointments: either they are fully cured and don't feel they need to come back, especially if they live in an insecure area or far from the facility; or they are dissatisfied with the result because they continue to leak. If a woman needs further care but can't or doesn't return for follow-up, there's not much we can do to help her, alas. We also cannot properly assess our own effectiveness in her case.

Overall, however, MSF's experience has been positive. Word has spread in the places where we work and hundreds of women come to MSF to get treatment every year. There are also a handful of other medical humanitarian organizations active in under-resourced areas. I know that suffering has been alleviated.

The need is still great, unfortunately, and only a fraction of the women who need surgery receive it. To prevent tens of thousands more women from experiencing fistulas every year and to help the roughly three million women now living with fistulas, much work remains. And most of that work should happen before the fistulas ever occur, starting with a concerted effort to provide access to emergency obstetric services to more women, wherever they live.

[i] WHO, "10 facts on obstetric fistula". 2014; http://www.who.int/features/factfiles/obstetric_fistula/en/

[ii] WHO, Department of Making Pregnancy Safer, "Obstetric Fistula: Guiding principles for clinical management and programme development," p. 6 & 7. 2006. http://whqlibdoc.who.int/publications/2006/9241593679_eng.pdf

[iii] Martin, Joyce A., MPH, et al., "Births: Final Data for 2012," National Vital Statistics Reports, Vol. 62, No. 9, p. 5. CDC, December 2013; http://www.cdc.gov/nchs/data/nvsr/nvsr62/nvsr62_09.pdf

[iv] The Society of Obstetricians and Gynaecologists of Canada, "A Labour of Loss: Obstetric Fistula," Accessed December 2014. http://iwhp.sogc.org/index.php?page=obstetric-fistula

STORIES FROM PATIENTS

Chantal, 18, Gitega, Burundi

"When I went into labor, I went to the closest health center. There, they told me that I needed to wait, that I wasn't yet ready to give birth.

I waited an entire day and then my water broke. They had me up on a gynecological table, but unfortunately, the nurse wasn't there. My caretaker went to find her and tell her to come and see me. She came and found the baby's head breaching. She didn't do much to help—she couldn't really, because it was already too late.

They referred me to a hospital, and we went there on a motorcycle, the baby's head still breaching. They told us that they didn't have the proper supplies and equipment to deal with the situation, so they referred us to another hospital. Again we went. There they examined me and told me that the baby had died.

They tried to remove the baby by pushing on my belly, but that did not work. They had to do an episiotomy and use forceps and a ventouse to remove the baby. They gave the body to my husband. He went to find a place for the burial. Since then, my husband hasn't come to see me.

I was leaking urine, so once I arrived back home, I went to the local health center. There they told me that they couldn't do anything about such a problem.

They called for an ambulance to come and take me to Mukenge hospital. The ambulance came, but when I got to Mukenge, they said they couldn't treat this problem either. We should call MSF in Gitega, they said, because their Urumuri health center has the capacity to deal with it.

They called the Urumuri center and I spoke to someone there. She said

'Go get a ticket for transport, come to Gitega and we will reimburse you.' It wasn't easy to get the money together—my father had to rent a small piece of his land.

I got a warm welcome at the Urumuri center. Now I'm waiting to see what happens, whether I'll need surgery or if the fistula will heal on its own. I feel good here, aside from having this problem. I am able to walk, even if I have pains in my right leg. I get along with the other women here; we are all suffering from the same thing and we can talk about it together."

Monique, 37, Kabezi, Burundi

"I have been pregnant nine times, but I gave birth for the first time last Friday. My first pregnancy was in the year 2000. I was in labor for a long time, and there was a lot of confusion and chaos.

I was supposed to give birth naturally, but in the end, the baby died. Since then, I've had incontinence [*the result of an obstetric fistula*] and I have been unable to carry a child to term. It was terrible not to be able to have a baby. It was a desperate feeling. I saw a number of doctors to try to have the fistula repaired. Eventually I was able to have repair surgery during a fistula camp.

My latest pregnancy was fine, but my water broke five days ago, at 29 weeks. When I felt it happen, I immediately started to cry. My first thought was that the baby is going to die. That's what happened last time and I lost my child.

I went to the health center near me in Mutambo when it happened, and I told them how many miscarriages I've had. They said to wait there and called the ambulance from MSF's center in Kabezi to come and get me. When I arrived at the facility, they operated on me right away. They gave me a C-section. I was desperate. All I wanted to do was to see my baby, to make sure he was still alive.

When he was born, he was so tiny. He weighed so little. Every day he seems to get better, which gives me hope. The doctors, too, give me hope that he'll live.

The local health centers around here don't seem to have the necessary resources to take care of women in labor. I get the impression that most of them call out to the Kabezi health center for an ambulance to come and pick the women up, which can obviously take time. And what about the urgent cases?

I have to thank my husband for sticking with me and having supported me in all this. He has been with me during all these miscarriages. He has been with me even when I was leaking urine. He's helped me to go get care when I needed it in Bujumbura. He's never left me, despite the fact that plenty of people in our circle have told him to.

I am so, so happy to be a mother. There really aren't any words. To be a parent, it's an immense pleasure that I can't even describe. Since my baby was born I've felt my mood lift."

Divine, 20, Gitega, Burundi

"Not long ago, I was pregnant with my first child. I started experiencing pains in my abdomen, so I asked someone to accompany me to the nearest health center, which is two hours away on foot.

When I arrived at the health center, they told me that despite the pains, it wasn't yet time for me to give birth. I waited two days and the baby still wasn't coming, so they transferred me to the Kirundo hospital. They examined me at the hospital and found that the baby had died.

It was really hard when I lost the baby. What's more is that I could have died too. I had an infection in my abdomen after the Caesarean section they gave me. I had to return to the hospital for the doctors to re-open the incision and clean out the inside. I spent another month at the hospital before I could go home.

People from my village kept asking what was wrong with me, why I was leaking urine all the time. I couldn't tell them what the problem was because I didn't know. So I just stayed at home, sad—I didn't leave the house. I didn't talk about it to anyone, except a community health worker who came to visit the village.

When I told her my story, we went to the closest health center. There, I was told that what I had was a fistula, and that I could get this problem treated in Gitega [*at MSF's Urumuri center*]. I explained all this to my family, and we got together some money to pay the price of transport. When I arrived here, I felt very well taken care of. I was given what I'd need and was shown where I would sleep. I still leak urine because I haven't had the procedure to fix it yet. But I'm waiting for the operation and I believe that it will work.

I feel good now, and I'm no longer unhappy. There's a really good atmosphere here. My husband comes to see me here often. My family and members of my church come to visit too.

To aid the healing process after the operation, there are recommendations that patients are supposed to follow, like refraining from sexual relations for three months. They seem a bit difficult. I agree with all of them but I don't know if my husband will accept them. I don't really know what I'll do if that's the case.

In order to stop this sort of thing happening to other women, I think they should avoid having children too young. I think they should study first, and then have kids. I wasn't able to go to school when I was young, but if I had, I would have continued my studies and probably would not have become pregnant so soon in life. I hope my children will all go to school and become nuns and priests, or health care workers."

CHAPTER 4

"There Is No Abortion Here" The Consequences of Unsafe Abortion

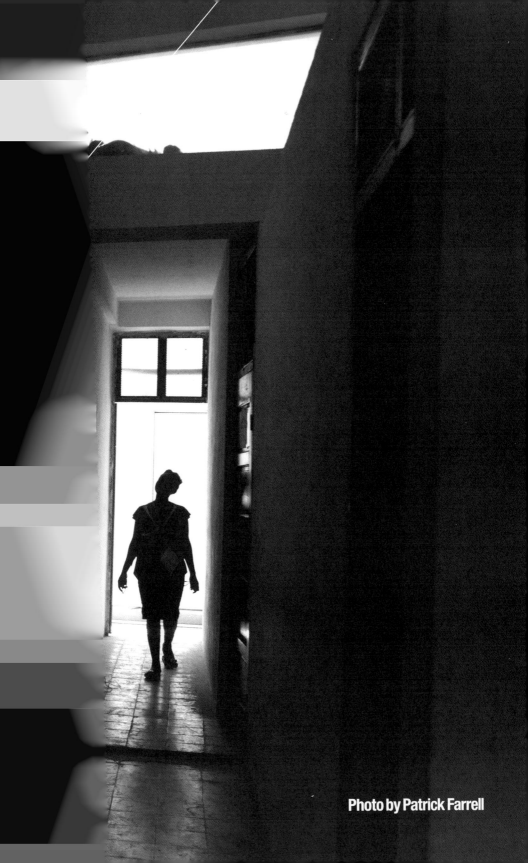

Photo by Patrick Farrell

Chapter 4
"There Is No Abortion Here" The Consequences of Unsafe Abortion

By Séverine Caluwaerts, OBGYN, MPH,
with Catrin Schulte-Hillen, Midwife, MPH

It was late at night when the staff called me to the hospital. Julie, one of our colleagues, had arrived, bleeding severely and shivering with a high fever. She was lying on a blood-soaked bed and was white as a sheet.

Four days earlier Julie had come to me, begging for help. She was an excellent midwife. She worked beside me at an MSF project in what I will call Country A. We were always busy, and whenever she was in the labor ward, I knew she would take very good care of the mothers and their babies.

She was only 24, but she seemed older and more mature. During breaks, we would drink tea and talk about our families and our work. She told me that she was supporting her three younger sisters so they could finish their studies.

I was completely unprepared one morning when Julie came to me in tears and whispered that she needed to see me privately. I poured her a cup of tea and she told me her story. For a few months she had been seeing a man who at first had not told her he had a wife and two children.

They had used condoms initially, but her partner preferred not to use them and contraception was not easy to get, especially for an unmarried woman. Since everyone knew everyone else in the community, it was difficult for Julie to go to the pharmacy to buy condoms or birth control pills. People would consider her promiscuous, a "bad girl."

Like millions of women before and after her, Julie became pregnant at the wrong time with the wrong person. Hers was an unplanned pregnancy. She had told her partner two days earlier but had not heard back from him.

In Country A, religion has a strong influence on policy. An unmarried pregnant woman is looked at with a scorn that extends to her family and community.

"This is the worst thing that has ever happened to me, Dr. Séverine," she told me. "I can never tell my family because it will bring so much shame upon them."

Abortion is legally restricted in Julie's country, even in the case of rape. The only legal exception for termination of pregnancy is to save the life of the mother. This is the case in 66 countries. In 71 others, the state has additional provisions for abortion if, for instance, they preserve the woman's mental or physical health or are being sought for certain socioeconomic reasons. Fifty-six nations place no restrictions, while three ban it unconditionally and entirely.[i]

Our project in Country A had only recently opened. We had not yet assessed the possible repercussions for women, staff, and the project if we were to provide abortion care. We still needed to take into account what the community would say and whether it would affect our ability to work in the area. The broader political situation there was not stable. Our headquarters had therefore decided that we could not perform abortions.

Julie was crying. I told her: "I want to help you, but as you know we do not do abortions in this project." I also asked if she had a trustworthy person in her life with whom she could discuss the situation.

"No," she said, "you are the only one who can help me."

Julie knew that MSF had the drug misoprostol, which is used to induce abortions, because we used it in that project to treat postpartum hemorrhages. She asked if there was any way I could get her some tablets, but I told her that I could not.

I struggled with this decision—my medical duty was to help her; I respected her decision to have an abortion for reasons of her own, and I wanted more than anything to do something for her, but doing what she asked in this case could have had severe repercussions for Julie and the project. MSF could have been expelled from the country, leaving it unable to help thousands of people in need. If we had been in another country in a calmer time and our headquarters had approved it, we could have provided the abortion ourselves or referred her to a safe provider, as we do in other places. But there were no safe referral options that we were aware of.

Julie did not say anything else. I asked her to return in a week's time and was hoping, in vain, that this unwanted pregnancy would perhaps become a miscarriage. I did not expect that when I saw her next I would be trying to save her life.

I examined Julie. Her cervix was open and foul-smelling contents were leaking out. She urgently needed a blood transfusion and antibiotics. Once they were administered, we brought her to the operating theater so we could remove the remaining septic matter.

With no other recourse, Julie had sought an abortion from someone with no medical training. I suspected that whoever performed the procedure had used a dirty rod to dilate her cervix in a crude attempt to induce the abortion. In doing so they had put Julie's life in jeopardy.

But Julie was lucky. She had a nearly fatal septic abortion but got treatment and recovered in a few days. I told her colleagues that she was admitted for a blood transfusion and antibiotics. I'm sure they suspected the unsafe abortion, but no one asked. Perhaps it was female solidarity; the other local midwives and staff certainly had daughters, sisters, or female friends who had been confronted with the same problem. To my knowledge, her partner did not visit her during her recovery.

The immediate, life-threatening complications from unsafe abortions are profuse bleeding, infection, and perforation of the uterus and adjoining organs. If the woman or girl survives, lifelong suffering, including chronic pelvic pain and infertility, can ensue. The human cost—suffering and often death—that women and girls bear alone at home after unsafe abortions is enormous, as is the suffering caused by the consequences of an unwanted pregnancy. Much of this cannot be measured with statistics.

But we do know that of the roughly 44 million abortions that occur every year, around half are unsafe, meaning they are performed by persons lacking the necessary skills or they occur in an environment lacking minimal medical standards, or both.[ii] These are only the abortions that are reported. The vast majority of unsafe abortions occur in developing countries in Africa and Latin America, as well as in China and Eastern Europe.[iii]

We also know that unsafe abortion is one of the five main causes of maternal mortality worldwide, together with hemorrhage, eclampsia, sepsis, and obstructed labor. Unsafe abortion accounts for a shocking 13 percent of maternal deaths around the world, according to the World

Health Organization (WHO).[iv] The rates are even higher in certain regions, such as Latin America, and in contexts such as refugee camps and conflict areas.

There is a growing appreciation of the public health cost of managing the complications of unsafe abortion, a cost that is in economic terms much higher than the provision of safe abortion care.[v] The economics aren't often considered, but they play an important role in the dynamics of abortion.

On the one hand, it costs more to treat women who've had unsafe abortions; on the other, there is a market for both safe and unsafe abortions in legally restricted environments. Those who benefit have little interest in changing the laws. Either way, abortion is provided whether or not it is legally restricted. And in most cases, the less money the patient has, the less likely she is to have a safe abortion.

Some countries have concluded that severe legal restrictions on abortion do nothing to stop demand, and that the resulting public health tragedies hit low-income women the hardest and cost public health systems the most. Six years after South Africa liberalized its abortion law, deaths from unsafe abortion dropped by at least half, and the number of post-abortion complications fell dramatically. Pregnancy-related deaths in Nepal also dropped when abortion was legalized in 2004. Hospitalizations and deaths from unsafe abortions ended almost immediately after the United States legalized abortion in 1973.[vi]
This isn't to say that legalizing abortion solves everything. Social norms do not change overnight, stigmas endure, and shortages of skilled professionals often remain.

MSF's policy toward abortion is clear. We consider access to safe abortions to be a medical necessity—an important and lifesaving part of comprehensive reproductive health care that reduces maternal mortality and prevents unsafe abortions. In fact, unsafe abortion is the only cause of maternal mortality that is entirely preventable.

On a daily basis, MSF staff in hospitals and emergency rooms the world over see women and girls with complications from unsafe abortions brought in for treatment. They come in pain and are often ashamed, intimidated, and afraid of the staff's reaction to what they've done. Some come bleeding and frightened; the person who sold them pills on the street or in a shop didn't tell them what to expect when they tried to abort. For these patients, counseling, medical information, and discussion of future contraceptive options might be enough. Others arrive with life-threatening bleeding, severe infections, perforated uteruses, or in septic shock. They require immediate medical care, and sometimes surgeries and blood transfusions, to save their lives.

To be clear, MSF has no desire to perform abortions just for the sake of it. Rather, MSF wants to make sure women have access to safe abortions, carried out by trained medical staff, in order to keep women from the suffering and death that result from unsafe abortions. Ideally, unwanted pregnancies would be reduced, but that aim would depend on removing restrictions placed on the availability and discussion of contraception in many places. If Julie or others like her had been able to access a method of contraception that corresponded to her needs, she may not have gotten pregnant in the first place, and would not have then risked a procedure that nearly killed her.

During my time in Country A, many women came in following what I believed were unsafe abortions. Some were infected and near death. But when I asked, they always denied that they had tried to terminate their pregnancy. The stigma was too great.

This was in 2009; the project in Country A closed in 2013 and never did provide abortions because of security concerns. During that time, however, making safe abortion care available has increasingly become a priority for MSF.

When I was the OBGYN in Bo, Sierra Leone, a 17-year-old girl named Fatmata was brought to the hospital. A schoolteacher had impregnated her. I was told that it was quite common for male teachers to molest or rape female students.

Fatmata told her mother and grandmother what had happened and the family decided together to go to a traditional birth attendant (TBA) to end the pregnancy and avoid the shame that would befall the family were she to carry the baby to full term. The TBA performed an unsafe abortion with an iron rod. The pregnancy was terminated, but the TBA also perforated the wall of Fatmata's uterus and made a hole in the bowel, a common result of unsafe abortions.

By the time they reached the hospital, Fatmata's mother thought her daughter was going to die. She had a fever of 102° F (39° C) and was suffering severe abdominal pain. An ultrasound revealed an infected mass of around 10 cm.

We gave Fatmata painkillers and antibiotics and referred her immediately to a project in the capital, Freetown, run by Emergency, an Italian aid agency with very capable surgeons. They resected part of Fatmata's bowel, but because her abdomen was so infected, they needed to perform a colostomy.

The result of this unsafe abortion was a 17-year old girl who had endured physical and emotional trauma and was left with a possibly permanent stoma. She may also have been rendered infertile. Even if she was not, any future pregnancies will come with a high risk of being ectopic (implanted outside of the uterus) and life-threatening.

Despite MSF's clear policy that safe abortion should be integrated as part of reproductive health care in all contexts where it is relevant, MSF cannot provide abortions in every project for every patient who requests one. Few of our projects, in fact, provide termination of pregnancy on request. Doing so could endanger patients and staff, given the legal context and the communities' perceptions of abortion in a given country. There are voices within MSF who want to reconsider this policy, however, and who stress that while weighing the risks to MSF personnel, we should also consider the risk facing the girl or woman—who we know will get an abortion one way or another.

Where MSF makes termination of pregnancy available, the staff will provide the service until the end of the first trimester. At a later gestational age, it is considered on a case-by-case basis. When a competent provider is accessible, we'll refer patients to avoid duplicating services.

MSF's treatment protocol favors medical abortion and manual vacuum aspiration. A medical abortion is the termination of pregnancy by administered drug. The combined use of mifepristone with misoprostol is effective in early pregnancy and is much less invasive than surgical procedures such as dilation and curettage (D&C) or vacuum aspiration. But it takes time. While D&C can only be performed by a physician in most countries, manual vacuum aspiration can be performed by other health staff, including midwives, and it is immediate. The choice of which procedure to use depends on the context and the medical condition of the patient. If all things are equal, the patient should be offered the choice.

Misoprostol has become more widely available on the private market in many countries. In fact, it's a flourishing business for those who sell the drug where abortion is legally restricted. For girls and women in need of an abortion, it is much less dangerous than using a metal rod or the other dreadful tools of unsafe abortion. But misoprostol is still risky for a woman or girl without having a medical assessment, as well as information on how to use the drug, what to expect after taking it, and what warning signs to look for. She also misses out on follow-up care, including contraception counseling and access to effective contraception for as long as she needs to suppress fertility.

At the Conference on Population and Development in Cairo two decades ago, the international community acknowledged the reality of maternal mortality and agreed that it could not be remedied unless contraceptives and safe abortion care were provided to women and girls, alongside safe obstetric care. Since then, much work has gone into providing or advocating for skilled obstetric care in developing countries, but the opposition remains adamant in the very countries where the highest numbers of women are dying from unsafe abortions.

Speaking with local health staffs, national health authorities, and political decision makers in many countries, I find they are generally sensitive to the medical arguments for the need to provide safe abortion care. But people frequently insist that unsafe abortions are something that does not happen in their community.

"We do not have this problem," I have been told. "Our women are religious; there is no abortion done here."

All the evidence points to the opposite conclusion: that women and girls will risk unsafe abortions to terminate unwanted pregnancies if no safe abortion care is available—even if they know the life-threatening risks, even if abortion is against the law, and even if community leaders deny that it is occurring. Julie was a midwife, after all. She knew the risks but took the chance because the alternative was unbearable for her and those around her.

If countries and communities are serious about reducing maternal mortality, there must be a realistic discussion about unwanted pregnancies. People should recognize that most women are denied control over their sexual lives, and there should be a commitment to change that—through easy access to contraception.

Abortion is obviously a charged subject, but from a medical perspective and from MSF's work in emergency rooms around the world, it's clear that the provision of safe abortion care to a woman or girl is a life-saving medical act. As long as access to safe abortion care is denied, more women and girls like Julie and Fatmata will continue to suffer, and many more women and girls will continue to die each year from the consequences of unsafe abortion.

[i] Center for Reproductive Rights, "The World's Abortion Laws Map." Last modified September 17, 2014. http://reproductiverights.org/en/document/the-worlds-abortion-laws-map

[ii] Susan A. Cohen, "Access to Safe Abortion in the Developing World: Saving Lives While Advancing Rights." Guttmacher Policy Review, 15, No. 3. Fall 2012. http://www.guttmacher.org/pubs/gpr/15/4/gpr150402.html

[iii] WHO, "Unsafe Abortion: Global and Regional Estimates of the Incidence of Unsafe Abortion and Associated Mortality in 2008." Sixth edition. P. 18-26. 2011. http://whqlibdoc.who.int/publications/2011/9789241501118_eng.pdf?ua=1

[iv] Sneha Barot, "The Missing Link in Global Efforts to Improve Maternal Health." Guttmacher Policy Review, 14, No. 2. Spring 2011. http://www.guttmacher.org/pubs/gpr/14/2/gpr140224.htm

[v] Michael Vlassoff, Damian Walker, Jessica Shearer, David Newlands and Susheela Singh, "Estimates of Health Care Systems Costs of Unsafe Abortion in Africa and Latin America." Guttmacher Institute. 2009. http://www.guttmacher.org/pubs/journals/3511409.html

[vi] Susan A. Cohen, "Facts and Consequences: Legality, Incidence and Safety of Abortion Worldwide." Guttmacher Policy Review. 12, No. 4. Fall 2009. https://www.guttmacher.org/pubs/gpr/12/4/gpr120402.html

Saving Two Lives

Photos by Martina Bacigalupo
Kabezi, Burundi

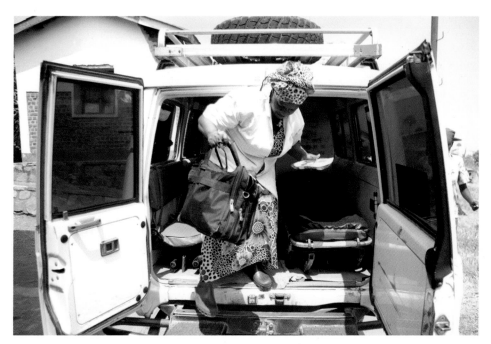

An MSF nurse arrives at Kabezi State Hospital.

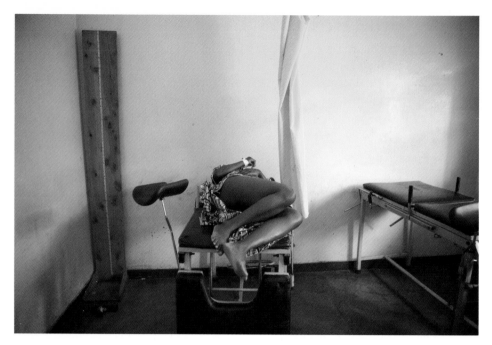

Chantal, 20 years old, is pregnant and in pain at the state hospital. The staff learned that she has had two Caesarean sections from previous pregnancies, which will put her at risk for uterine rupture if she tries to give birth vaginally. She needs surgical care, so the nurses called the MSF hospital.

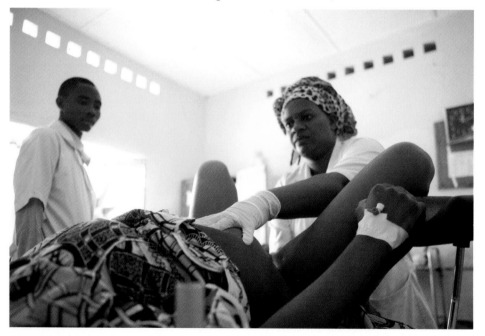

The MSF nurse examines Chantal and stabilizes her for the journey to the MSF hospital.

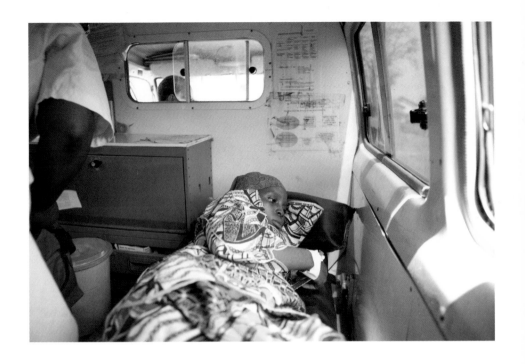

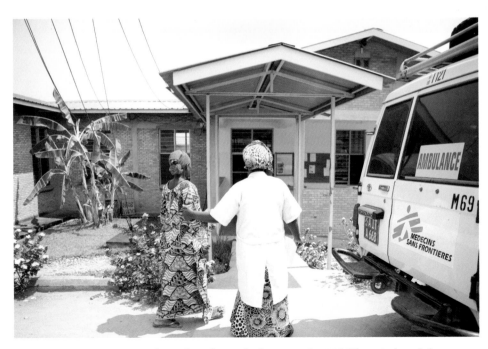

The nurse accompanies Chantal in the ambulance to the MSF hospital and then helps her inside.

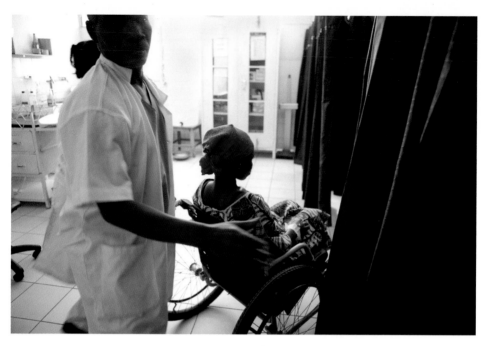

Chantal's baby is in a breech position and there are signs that her uterus might rupture. She is prepared for immediate delivery by Caesarean section.

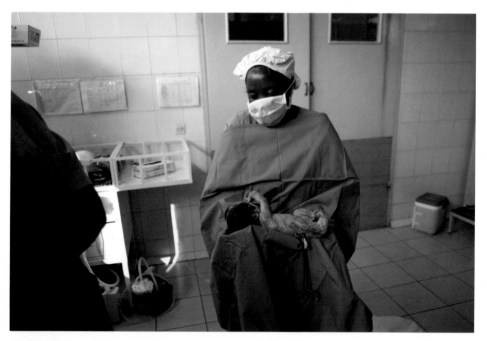

A baby boy is delivered and the midwife attends to him.

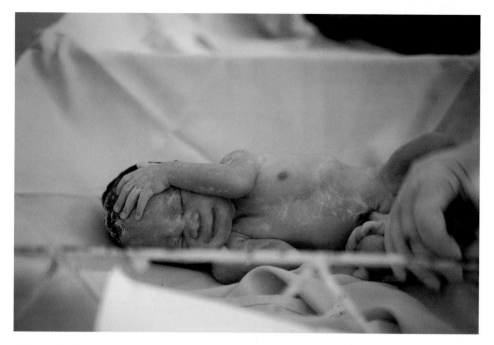

Although Chantal's newborn son is premature, he weighs nearly five pounds and is otherwise healthy.

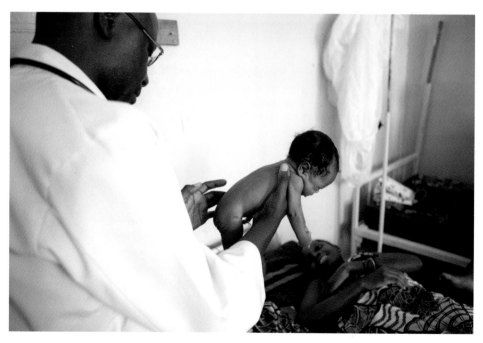

An MSF doctor checks in on the newborn and his mother.

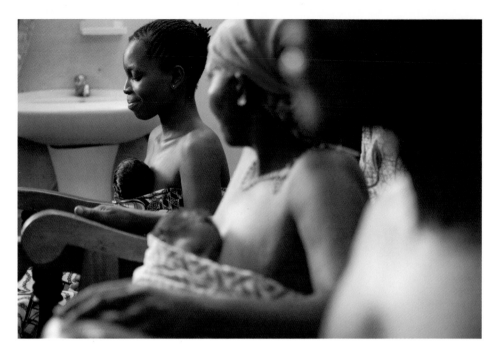

Chantal learns "kangaroo care," in which the baby is pressed to the mother's chest for warmth, bonding, and breast milk stimulation, and joins other mothers in the "kangaroo room."

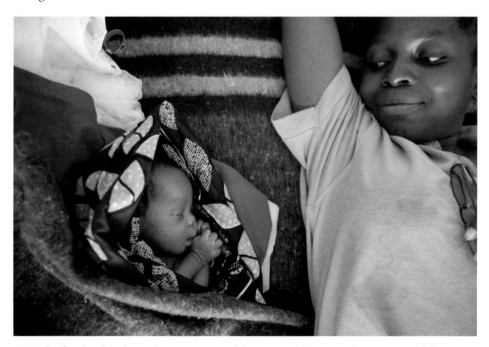

A week after birth, Chantal's son is out of the neonatal unit and can stay with her. When both are strong and healthy, they will go home.

A Second Chance

Photos by Martina Bacigalupo
Gitega, Burundi

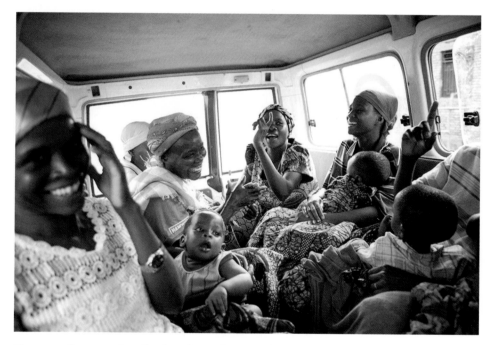

Yvonne, 48, center, has lived with an obstetric fistula for 22 years. Today she and several other women are on their way to receive fistula repair surgery at MSF's Urumuri Center in Gitega.

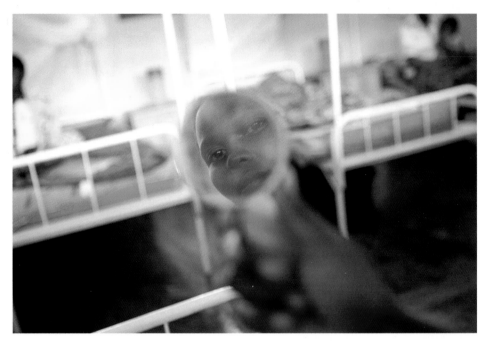

Evelyne, 23, waits on the day of her surgery at the Urumuri Center. She developed a fistula during her second delivery, on a roadside, while trying to reach a hospital.

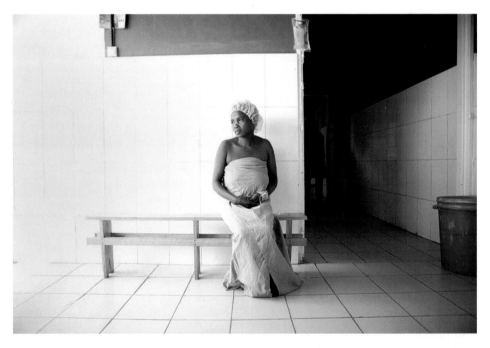

Yvonne nervously awaits her operation. She sustained a fistula when she delivered her first baby at home.

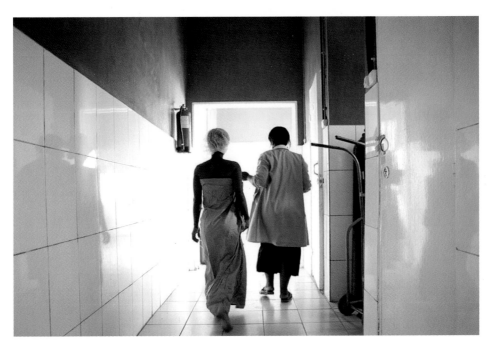

A nurse leads Evelyne to the operating room. A week after her surgery, she will begin daily exercises to regain bladder control. In order to heal successfully, she will need to stick to a strict post-operative care regimen for up to six months.

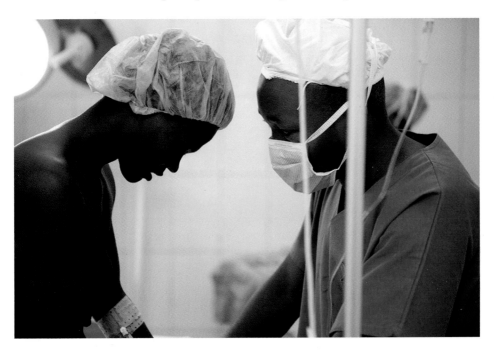

One of the doctors tries to help Evelyne relax before surgery.

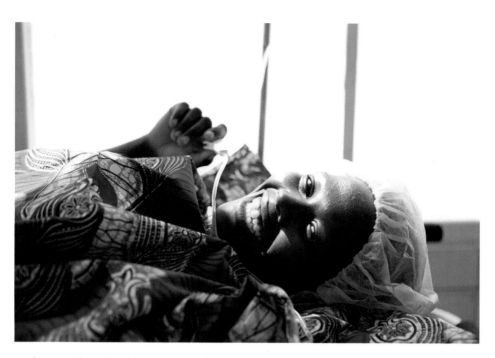

Evelyne smiles when the surgery is over.

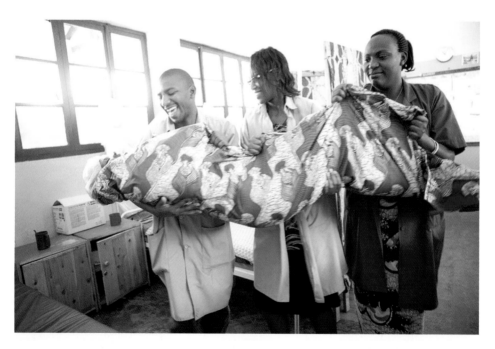

Nurses move Evelyne from the gurney onto her bed.

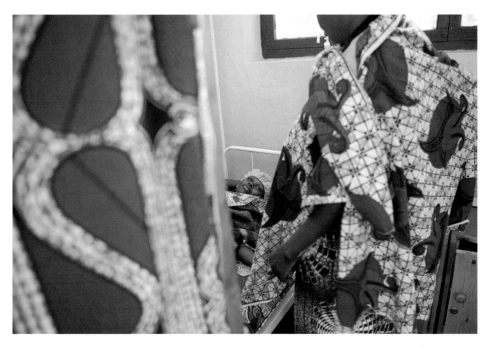

Yvonne, who received surgery a week before, pays Evelyne a visit.

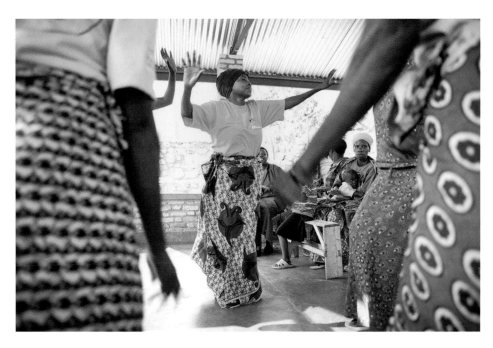

During the last days of her stay, Yvonne dances with fellow patients.

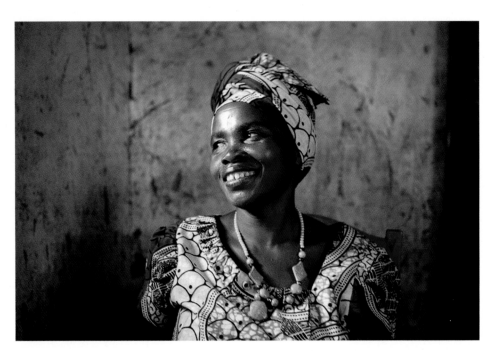

Yvonne smiles, back home after her fistula repair surgery. She says she wants to help spread the word about the availability of treatment. "Many women hide their problems and die, when they could be saved," she says.

Delivering HIV-Free

Photos by Sydelle Willow Smith
Thyolo, Malawi

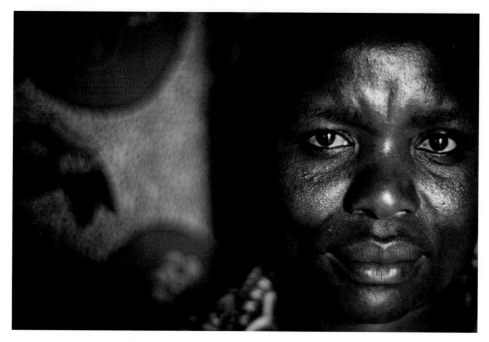

Edna is a patient in the prevention of mother-to-child transmission of HIV (PMTCT) program in Thyolo. "When they told me [that I was HIV-positive], I was very worried and afraid," she says. "I was only going to the clinic to find out if I was pregnant and not to be hearing this kind of news. I thought, 'How am I going to tell my husband about this? What if he tells me this is the end of our marriage?'"

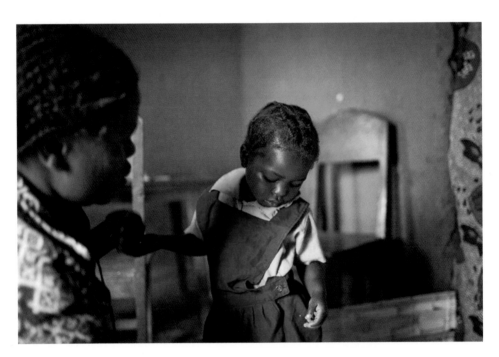

Edna dresses her daughter at home in Thyolo. Edna's husband left her for a short time, but then came back. They worked together to keep their baby from becoming HIV-positive.

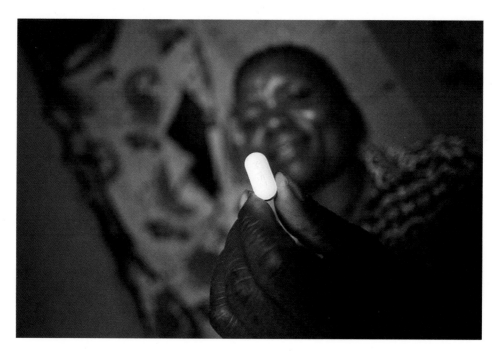

Edna holds up one of her antiretroviral pills. It took time for her to deal with the reality that she would be on medication for the rest of her life: "I knew it was a fact, but I had questions. Am I really going to take this all my life? How long is all my life? How about my children? Am I going to be healthy and still take care of them? What if I stop? What if I run out of medicine? I took all these questions to counseling with the peer mothers. They helped me feel strong."

Peer mothers are women who have been through the PMTCT program already and can help counsel newly enrolled mothers during the challenges of treatment.

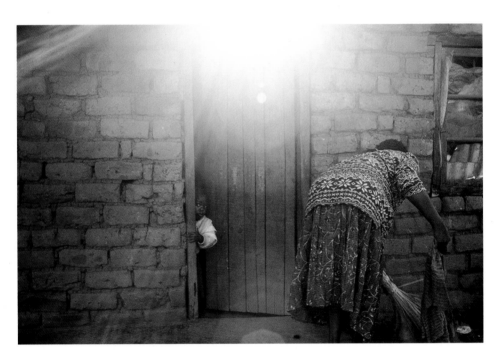

Edna sweeps while her daughter watches. When her daughter turned two years old, Edna took her for her final HIV test and the child was declared HIV-free. "They told me, 'Your child is definitely negative. Thank you for your great work and care of this baby.' I was extremely happy when they told me that."

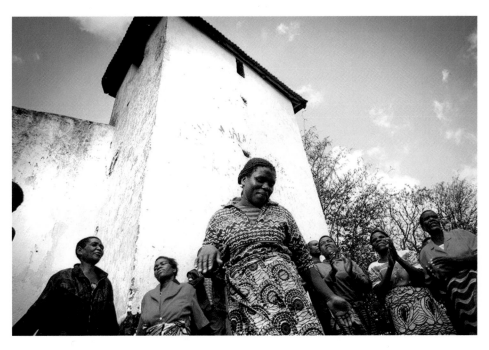

Edna, like many mothers in PMTCT programs, has benefited greatly from both individual counseling and community support groups.

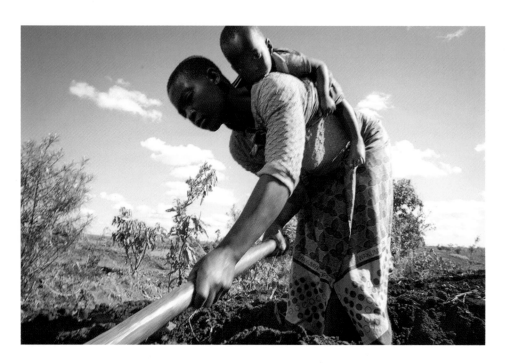

Jennipher is also a PMTCT patient in Thyolo. She and her husband discovered they were HIV-positive when she was pregnant for the third time, with twins. "When my husband was around we were living happy. We were farming. My husband could tell when I was tired and he would tell me that I could go back home while he finished the farming. Then I would come home and prepare a meal for him."

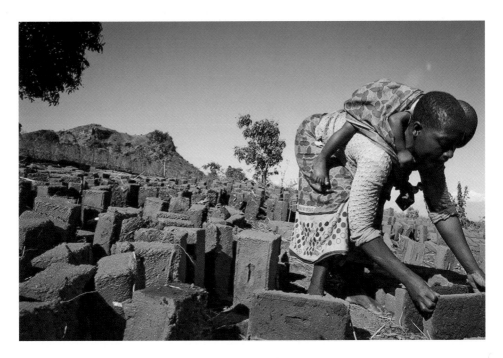

"When I got pregnant the last time, we went together as husband and wife to the first antenatal visit. We both got tested and they told us we were both HIV-positive. He insisted he was not sick and would not get treatment." Jennipher and her husband attended marriage counseling, but things did not improve.

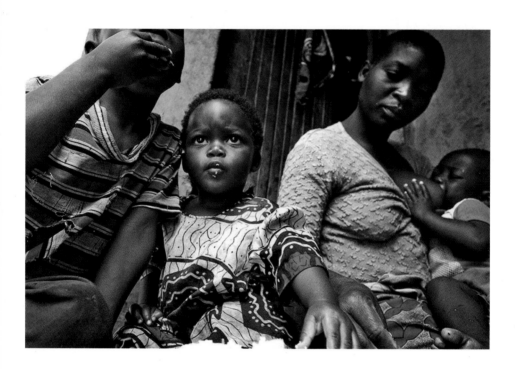

Jennipher supports and cares for her four children by herself now. "My husband
didn't leave me with any money. I was worried what about what I was going to do
with these children, where I was going to get money to buy food for them. I felt abandoned. I was crying sometimes."

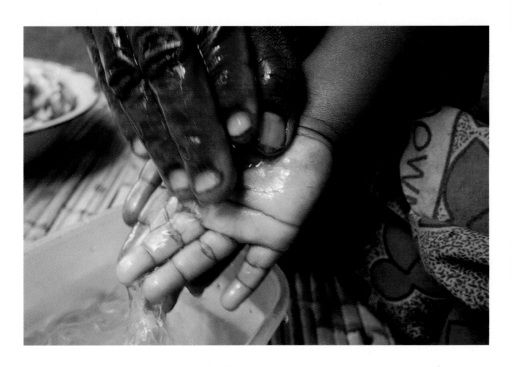

Jennipher washes her baby's hands after the meal.

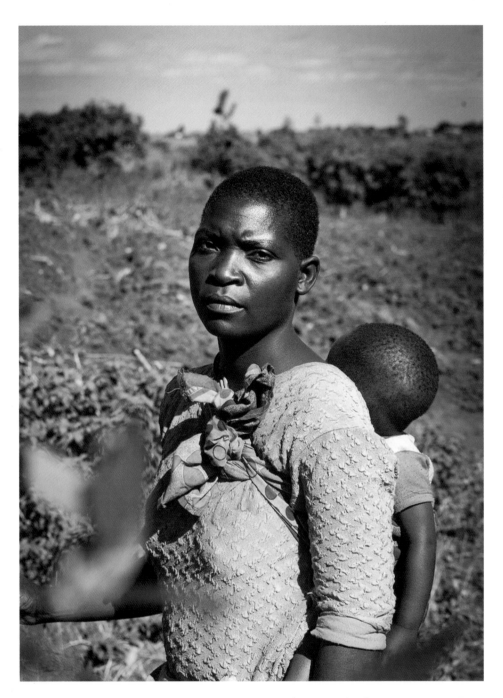

"I get the support I need from the peer mothers. Ever since the first visit, I've made sure that every time I go to the clinic, I see them. Even if they're busy with other women, I wait and make sure I meet with them. I was able to leave my worries aside because I got enough encouragement from these women."

"Tari Women Are Very Strong"

Photos by Kate Geraghty
Tari, Papua New Guinea (PNG)

"Tari women can make their own garden,
sell things at the market, and keep pigs. They can divorce
their husbands and raise the kids by themselves if
the husband is not supporting the family. Some are sad and
they struggle to survive. But in general, Tari women are
very strong." – Leonie, national staff counselor

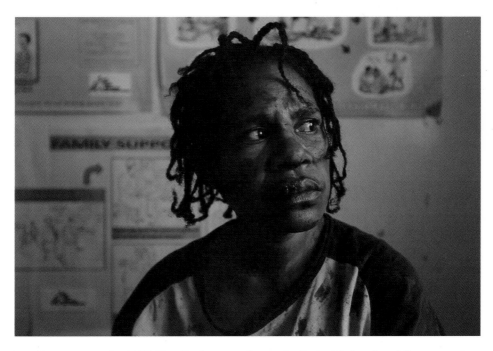

Marilyn came to the MSF Family Support Center in Tari with head and face wounds
after being beaten by her husband and his new wife. Many patients at the center have
been wounded by husbands, co-wives, or other relatives.

In Tari, an impoverished town in the rural Southern Highlands of PNG, MSF's Family Support Center offers medical and mental health care to survivors of family and sexual violence, both of which are very common in PNG. MSF's presence in that country is unique. Although the organization treats patients for trauma in many of its projects, only in PNG does it specifically reach out to victims of family and domestic violence.

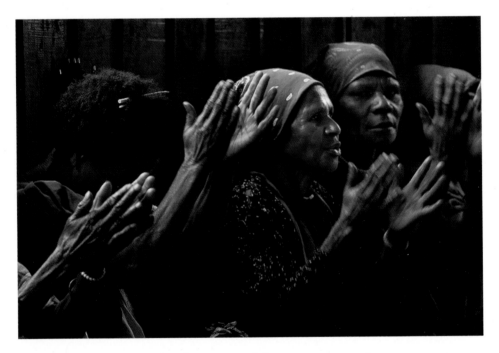

Women pray and sing in church. "To stop violence, we try to get boys to come to church," says one patient. "I have a son. I would like him to be a doctor. I will talk to my son and tell him not to hit women and not to kill men and not to steal."

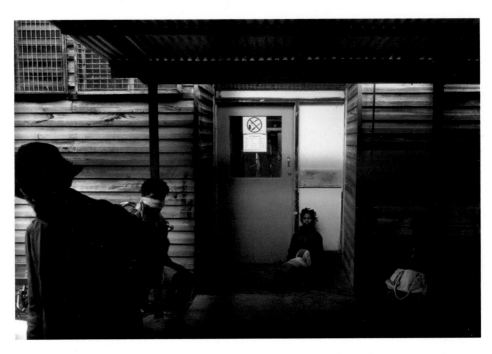

Patients wait outside the minor operation room. Treating physical injuries is often the easy part. Because patients face problems larger than fractures and wounds, medical care is integrated with mental health counseling.

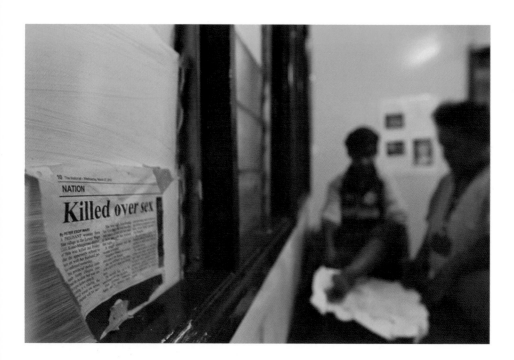

A newspaper clipping hangs on a wall inside the center. "There have been media reports and members of parliament have discussed giving harsher penalties to rapists and people who are violent against family members," says Leonie, a national staff counselor. "But nothing has happened yet."

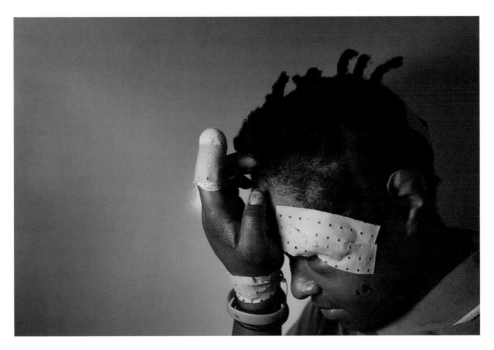

Marlin came to the Family Support Center after her husband attacked her with a machete. "He really frightens me. I'm going to die. That's really how I felt," she says.

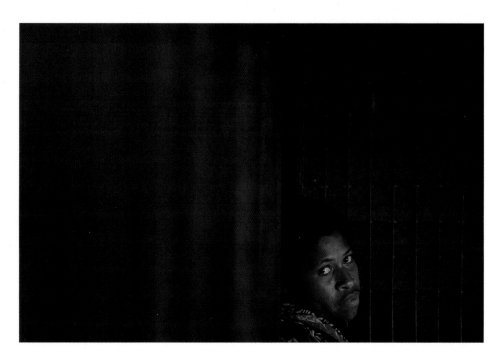

"Four days after we were married," says Josephine, a patient, "my husband's co-wife stabbed me. At the MSF clinic after the operation, I thought I had died and come back to life again. If she comes to Tari, she must know she is a dead woman. I am still angry. I'll make sure she gets a mark in the same place I got it. I don't think she'll come."

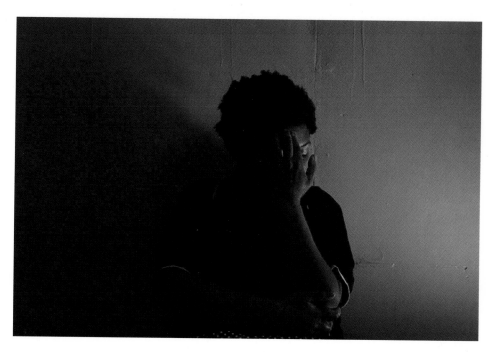

"The physical problem we could take care of," says an MSF doctor who treated Josephine, "but the bigger problem had not been solved. Now it was unsafe for her to go home. We offered counseling to discuss other ways of dealing with her anger."

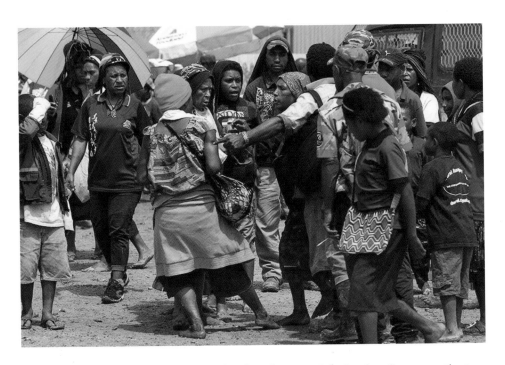

"My village always has problems. My brothers have [cut] their wives," says a patient named Tapali. "I get mad at them. Sometimes I tell the wives to divorce my brothers. I have taken them to MSF for treatment. I get scared [of the violence] sometimes and run away and hide."

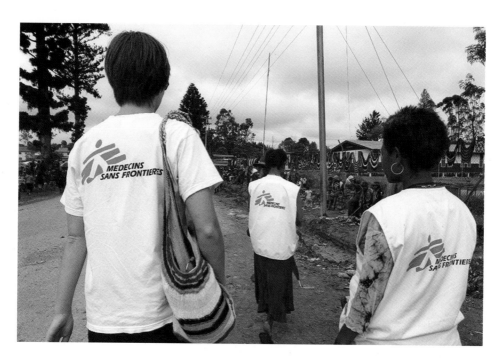

An MSF outreach team goes into town to let people know that care for sexual and family violence is available for free at MSF's Family Support Center.

No Good Choice

Photos by Patrick Farrell
Port-au-Prince, Haiti

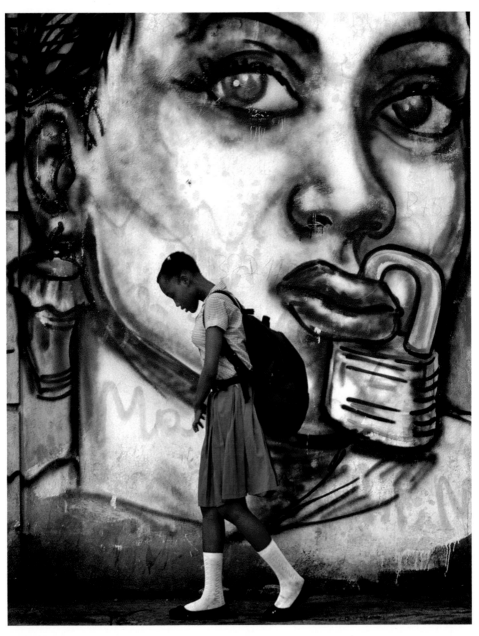

A student of a girl's school in Port-au-Prince walks by a mural depicting the suppression of women in Haiti, one of the 140 countries where abortion is legally restricted.

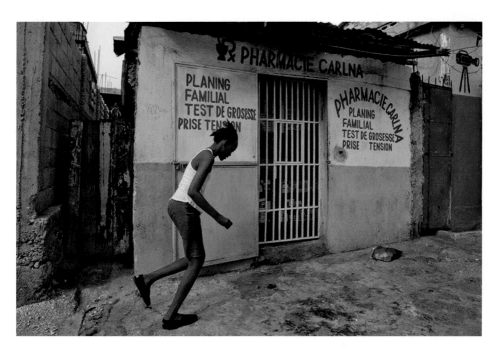

A girl plays outside a typical pharmacy in downtown Port-au-Prince where miso-prostol, a drug used to induce abortions, is illegally and readily available without a prescription. Women and girls are not given instructions from a medical professional on how much to take or what to expect, and they receive no follow-up care.

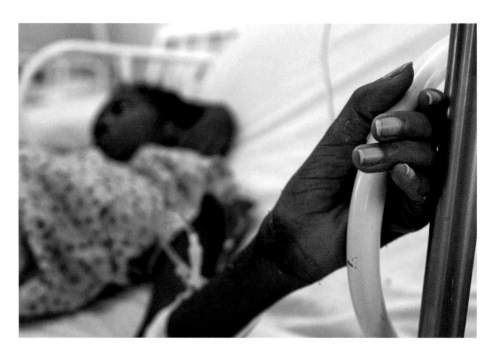

This 20-year-old woman arrived at MSF's hospital for obstetrical emergencies in Port-au-Prince suffering from a perforated uterus, excessive bleeding, and loss of fluids after an abortion performed by a non-licensed provider, known locally as a "charlatan." Thanks to prompt emergency treatment, she survived. Many others do not.

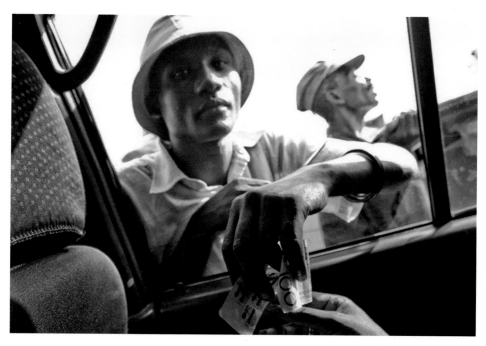

A street vendor sells Cytotec—a brand name of misoprostol—on the streets near the General Hospital in Port-au-Prince for the equivalent of $2.50. The pill is commonly used by women seeking to terminate their pregnancies.

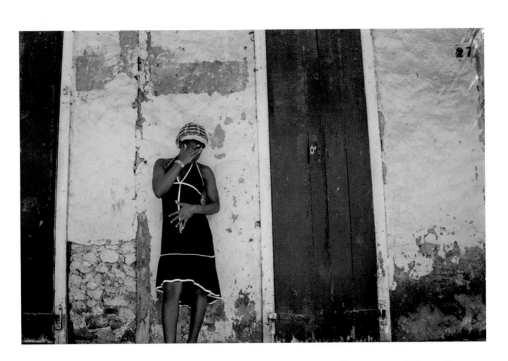

This 17-year-old girl from a rural town in Haiti is pregnant for a second time after she was repeatedly raped by a relative's husband. Her family does not believe her. She bought misoprostol off the street to terminate the first pregnancy when she was 16. Her choices this time are equally bleak.

CHAPTER 5

Treating Sexual Violence: A Long-Term Commitment

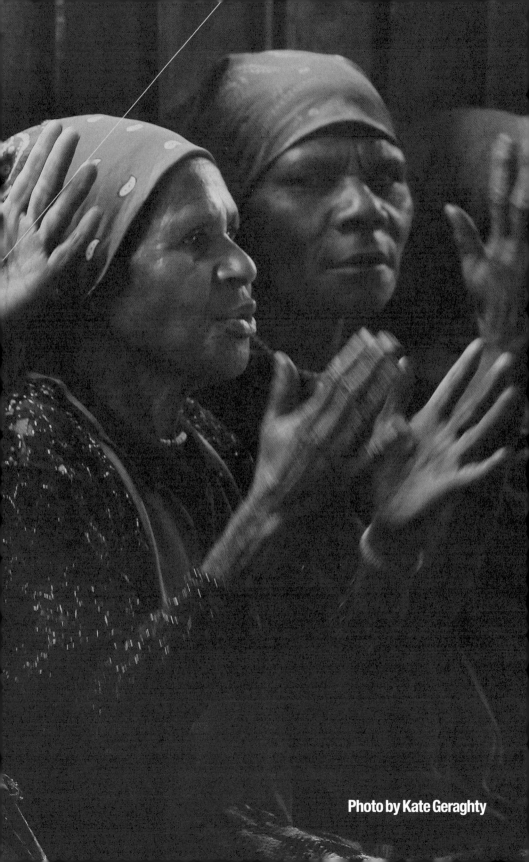

Photo by Kate Geraghty

Chapter 5
Treating Sexual Violence: A Long-Term Commitment

Women and Girls, Casualties of War

By Ann Van Haver, Midwife

Beatrice was one of the roughly 100,000 people who flocked to Mpoko camp in January 2014. Mpoko was the largest of several displacement camps scattered around Bangui, the capital of Central African Republic (CAR). Like many, Beatrice was trying to escape the violence of an ongoing civil war and find shelter for herself and her children.

She had a few items she'd brought with her from her home but little to eat. When she ran out of food, or the children's clothes got too dirty or torn, Beatrice would have to return home to fetch some essentials. In this lawless context, where armed men were everywhere, that meant taking a huge risk.

"I went back to my house to collect clothes for my children," she later told me. "I was inside, looking for the things I wanted to pack when I heard a knock on the door. I didn't dare to open it, and before I could hide, five armed men in military uniform entered the house. They asked where my husband was. I told them he was not there. They pointed guns at me and forced me to lie down. One after the other passed over [raped] me, while two others were pushing me down. Another one told me he would kill me if I shouted for help. After they had finished, they left the house. I felt very tired and lay down to sleep. After a few hours I came back to the camp."

For several days, Beatrice had been too ashamed and too frightened to tell anyone what had happened. Then she heard from "the people with the megaphones"—MSF's health promotion teams at Mpoko—that victims of sexual violence could come to the MSF hospital at the edge of the camp for treatment. That's where I met her.

Beatrice was not alone in her suffering. During my five-week assignment in CAR, I listened to 31 women describe being sexually assaulted and raped. This was not my first time hearing such accounts, but these women's stories shocked me. I recount them here because they are both hard to believe and distressingly familiar, because they must be heard and the acts condemned, and because it's important that people realize that the provision of medical care for victims of sexual violence, while crucial, is only the beginning of what they need.

MSF treated more than 11,000 victims of sexual violence in 34 countries in 2013. About 95 percent of our patients are women and girls; 5 percent are men and boys.

It is MSF's policy for all projects to offer medical care to victims of sexual violence (Women, men, and children all suffer from these attacks, but the vast majority of victims are women and girls. For the purposes of this book, we will be speaking mainly about them). In CAR, we were in a conflict zone, in a makeshift camp for internally displaced people. As in most conflict settings, our focus was on lifesaving activities, but within three weeks of building a hospital from wood, plastic sheeting and tents, we started a sexual violence program.

I hired and trained a midwife dedicated to treating sexual violence victims, and I recruited three other midwives whom we would supervise. The psychologist at the project hired and trained two female social workers to work in teams with the midwives and to spread the word about our services throughout the camp.

Health care providers can do a lot for patients who have been through sexual violence, although it often seems inadequate for someone who has undergone such trauma. We can treat injuries, prevent or treat infections, manage unwanted pregnancy, offer psychological support, and provide medical certificates.

Stigma and shame, along with fear of repercussions, keep many victims of sexual violence from seeking treatment, however. The path to care must be discreet. At Mpoko, our health promoters distributed small pieces of paper with a referral code to potential patients, who'd then bring it to a female health promoter stationed at the hospital gate. The promoter would escort the patient to the far corner of the hospital, where we had set up a tent that served as the sexual violence treatment area. (We later moved it to an even more isolated area with a fence around it.)

Women who have suffered sexual violence will often come to a medical facility hoping to receive drugs that will let them sleep or alleviate recurrent headaches, body pain, and anxiety. But painkillers or sleeping pills alone won't help them. A counselor, a midwife or a nurse will describe how the shock of the violence can cause these symptoms, and how psychosocial counseling can be of service.

The concept of counseling is often new to the people MSF treats. It is therefore extremely important to create an atmosphere in which a patient feels free to talk, to cry, or to be silent. We work to build that space by first explaining that everything that is said will remain confidential, that we will not tell her story to anyone else, and that we will not judge her. We state as fact that what she endured was not her fault and that we know that she didn't want this to happen.

Beatrice arrived on the first day we began offering sexual violence treatment in Mpoko. When she was brought in, we asked what had happened so that we could understand the chronology of events and give her proper counseling and treatment. Many victims are not able to tell us everything at first, and we do not pressure them. It can take great effort and courage to revisit these episodes. It can be helpful, but it can also bring back the trauma of the experience. For that reason we ask them to recount their story only once.

Before I began the medical exam, I explained what I was going to do. I asked her permission before each time I touched her. For a sexual violence victim to undress and be prodded by a stranger can be extremely painful and even re-traumatizing. We therefore we seek approval and involvement at every step of the process. This protocol applies to children as well. If a child victim does not want to be touched, the exam should never be forced.

We gave Beatrice vaccines for hepatitis B and tetanus and antibiotics to prevent sexually transmitted infections. She was still within the five-day window to receive the morning-after pill to protect her from pregnancy, but too late for HIV prophylaxis, which must be given within 72 hours. If a patient has indeed contracted HIV, MSF can offer HIV counseling and testing and connect the patient with HIV services.

"We were hiding in our house when the soldiers came to our area," Deborah told us. "The neighbors yelled 'RUN!' but we were too late.

Four heavily armed men were already at our doorstep. My husband hid under the bed, but I didn't have a place to hide. The men asked where my husband was. I told them he was not at home. The leader decided to rape me. One man forced me down with a knife on my throat. When the other man was on top of me and inside me, he looked aside and saw my husband under the bed. He shot him while he was still on top of me and then continued with me. The other man raped me after him, then they left me unconscious in the house."

Deborah was calm when she came in. She seemed resigned, but the impact of the assault was already apparent. She was having difficulty sleeping and was wrestling with a deep sense of shame. She did not give more details of her story. We asked her, as we ask all sexual violence patients, to return for follow-up sessions so we could continue our work together.

Another woman, Sylvia, who was 24, came in just hours after being attacked. She struggled to find words at first but eventually told us what had happened. She had been selling fruit to earn money. "The man told me I had to come to the [international forces] military camp by 6 p.m., to pick up the money for my fruit," Sylvia said. "At 6 p.m. it is dark and there are a lot of bandits around the base. The area around there is empty, with bushes. Three men jumped out of the bushes. They took me far away and forced me to have sex with them. They put it in my mouth, in my behind and in my vagina. I fainted. They left me by the side of the road, naked. Two kind people helped me to find my way to the IDP camp. My mother washed me."

We did not press her for more details, and we gave her the full medical package. We also installed a bed in our sexual violence tent, gave her food, and let her sleep for several hours. When she woke up, we again explained her treatment and her follow up appointments. A psychoso-

149

cial counselor walked her back to where her mother was.

In the days that followed, we watched Sylvia closely. She met with our counselors twice a week. Within a week she was able to function, to talk, even to smile now and then. But she was having flashbacks, sleep ing poorly, and was afraid to walk in the street.

Women in areas of conflict, where there is often a complete breakdown of order, are particularly vulnerable to sexual violence. The threats can come from anywhere: government security forces, rebel groups, militias, and criminal elements that operate with impunity.

If that isn't enough, rape is often used systematically as a tactic of war, to devastate individuals and communities. During the 1994 Rwandan genocide, between 100,000 and 250,000 women were raped in three-months.[i] During the Bosnian War, thousands of women were held in "rape camps" and brutalized repeatedly.[ii] In eastern Democratic Republic of Congo (DRC), where fighting has plagued the country for more than 15 years, around 1,100 rapes are reported *every month*, with an average of 36 women and girls being raped daily. These are just the reported figures; the real numbers are assumed to be much higher.[iii] In MSF facilities alone, teams have provided medical care to more than 54,000 victims of sexual violence in eastern DRC over the last decade.

Women and girls are vulnerable to rape in other contexts, too—and often similarly hesitant to seek assistance. In Morocco in 2010, MSF teams found that large numbers of female migrants and asylum-seekers from other parts of Africa who were trying to reach Europe needed treatment for sexual violence but were afraid to seek help. MSF and other civil society organizations lobbied the government to improve care for migrants. They also pressed European Union countries to address the effects of increasingly restrictive policies on migrants. In 2011, Morocco passed a law affirming that health care was a fundamental human right for everyone, including migrants.

As a medical organization, MSF's priority is delivering the targeted medical and mental health care that sexual violence victims need. In certain situations, though, we go beyond that, advocating for changes in policies and procedures that can help facilitate care for those who need it. Morocco was one example. Guatemala is another. In Guatemala City, where violent criminal gangs all too frequently prey on women and girls, many survivors neither report rape nor seek treatment. Those who do may face threats and intimidation.

As in Morocco, MSF has advocated on behalf of victims, working to make clear to the authorities, the medical community, and the public in general that sexual violence is a medical emergency and that women who've been sexually assaulted must have access to treatment. Teams have also worked with the government and the country's medical system to improve data collection and case recording.

In cases of sexual violence, MSF offers patients medical certificates. The documents confirm that the patient came to MSF health services and recount the patient's story and what the staff's findings were upon medical examination. They do not attempt to confirm or deny rape, but state the patient's account and conclude whether, upon medical examination, the wounds and the results of the physical examination are consistent with the assault as described by the victim. Only 10 of the 31 women we treated while I was in Mpoko wanted a medical certificate. In conflict areas like CAR, there is simply nothing in place to support victims of sexual violence who want to seek justice.

We offer them the certificates anyway in case they decide they want to press charges and there is the opportunity to do so in the future.

Medical confidentiality, including the safeguarding of medical files and certificates, is critical in treating sexual violence patients. Confidentiality could be compromised at many different points in the recording and storing of information. To prevent this, medical staff need to be trained on how patients should be identified and how much information about them is needed and recorded.

Beatrice was one of the few women I saw who wanted a medical certificate, but her more pressing concern, and that of many other women in Bangui, was how she would feed her family. Most of the women and girls had lost a husband or father and were solely responsible for the children in their families. The camp was not consistently providing food, and making sure their children could eat was a much more immediate worry than legal recourse. What further risks would she have to take?

At that time, MSF teams were conducting around 12,000 medical consultations per week and working to provide water and sanitation services in the camps in Bangui. We were often the only organization providing assistance. MSF repeatedly called on the international community to respond. CAR is still struggling with a complete breakdown of order, and as of late 2014, the UN and donor countries had still done little to address the situation.

Sexual violence spreads unchecked in situations like this, where the vulnerable can find little protection, where women and children are assaulted with impunity, and where the care that they need is too often beyond their reach.

A Scourge in "Stable" Places
By Rebecca M. Singer, RN, ND

It was towards the end of the day at our clinic in Lae, the second-largest city in Papua New Guinea (PNG), when Jennifer came in. She had been absolutely brutalized, beaten all over her body and badly wounded. Jennifer told us she had been gang raped at a bus stop in the middle of town. Six men had attacked her on her way home from work. She knew some of them.

We cleaned her wounds, gave her prophylaxis against pregnancy and HIV, and told her she needed to come back to continue the HIV medication. "I can't," she said, "I just can't." She was ashamed that such a thing had happened to her, and she was afraid. She didn't want any more trouble. She wanted to put the whole thing behind her.

We begged her to come back. Finally she gave us her phone number, and we gave her a ride to her destination. We tried to follow up with her, but we never saw her again.

Jennifer said she felt alone in her experience. But her injuries, mental trauma, and sense of shame are shared by millions of women and girls who have suffered rape or sexual assault around the world. And not just in war zones. MSF also works in so-called stable settings, places where there is no active conflict but sexual violence is still a constant threat. PNG is one such place. South Africa is another; according to a study released in 2011, in fact, more than one in four men in South Africa said they had committed rape.[iv]

There is limited information on rates of sexual violence in PNG. Research conducted by Papua New Guinea Medical Research Institute in 1994 is the most commonly cited. Fifty-five percent of the women in the study said they'd been forced into sex against their will, usually by men they knew. Half of the married women surveyed said their husbands used beatings or threats to force them into sex. Sixty percent of men in the study said they'd participated in gang rapes.[v] But—and here is where the similarity to war zones comes in—women and girls in PNG can only rarely access medical care for their injuries or risk of infection. There is also very little social or psychological support for mental trauma and few legal avenues through which the perpetrators might be brought to justice.

In 2010 and 2011, I spent five months working in Lae as the project coordinator of MSF's program for victims of sexual and family violence. It was a unique program for MSF, one of the very few projects that specifically reaches out to victims of family violence, along with victims of sexual assaults. People wounded in family violence constituted most of the cases we saw, though we also treated many women and children for sexual violence as well—2,894 in all, between 2007 and 2013.

During my assignment in Lae, I came to realize that managing the medical care for victims of rape is the easy part. It's everything that comes before and after that is so complicated. As Jennifer's story illustrates, follow-up is a constant problem that can have severe consequences if it does not happen. Post-exposure prophylaxis for HIV is a 28-day course of treatment, for instance. MSF has seen that if patients are given the entire course of drugs at once, only half of them will complete it, so we try to get victims to come in again. The patient also needs to come more than once for effective tetanus protection; patients with hepatitis B must come back for a second and third shot.

Most patients never return at all, though, and thus never finish their treatment. When possible, MSF uses community health workers to find patients who miss follow-up appointments and try to persuade them to come back. This works with some, but not all.

There are many reasons why women may not return for follow-up. In places such as DRC, travelling means risking getting robbed or even raped again. Women in rural areas, far from the nearest treatment facility, may have no access to transportation. Another reason stems from a lack of understanding about the importance of the care. The value of a woman's or girl's health and well-being are not seen as high enough to offset the cost of receiving this care—whatever that cost may be.

In any context, a rape victim faces the risk of being identified. A woman who is not pregnant and is making many trips to the hospital could be talked about, and the fear of stigma and its social repercussions could be a price she does not want to pay. It's hard enough convincing women to come in for treatment the first time. Asking for a second or third visit only compounds the difficulty, no matter how necessary we tell them it is.

Perhaps the strongest barrier to victims receiving care is the shame that is so closely linked to rape. This is something I see in the U.S. and in the field alike. It's global, this immobilizing feeling that somehow the victim caused the rape to happen and must bear the consequences. When I worked with MSF in Liberia, a patient told me, "If you've already had sex and consented once, there is no such thing as rape after that." I also heard, "Well, I've been raped before, so..." It was as if it happened once, the next time it wouldn't matter.

When I worked in Liberia, there was a night when a woman named Marie was brought to our clinic in very bad shape. She had been gang raped after she went out dancing with her friends. She told me her story: she worked as a prostitute but that particular night she was just out to have a nice time. Now she didn't want anyone to know what hap-

pened, she said, because in her neighborhood, prostitution was accepted but rape was shameful. What's more, like many survivors of sexual
violence in Liberia, Marie did not want to go to the police, either. This
was a common sentiment; I heard many Liberian women say that they
feared retribution should their attackers learn that their victims reported the crime, and that they feared the police themselves, too. In Liberia
(and in PNG, and other countries), women all too often were raped
again by the very policemen to whom they reported the initial crime!

Sex crimes against children also go unreported. Children make up
roughly half of the victims of sexual violence that MSF sees. In Lae,
half the rape survivors we saw were children; among girls the median
age was 13. In Liberia the figure was around 80 percent with a median
age of 13 for girls and 10 for boys.

Children often don't tell anyone about the crime because they are
afraid of what might happen to the perpetrator, who may be a parent
or neighbor. They may also be intimidated into keeping quiet. Family
members may not want to confront each other even when they know
what has happened, or they don't want to endure the stigma or the
prospect of inviting retribution against the attacker, who might be the
husband, brother or uncle, and also perhaps the breadwinner for the
family. We saw many families in Liberia and PNG who brought their
children in for medical care but wouldn't report the rape to authorities.

It can be very difficult to help remove a victim of sexual violence from
danger at home. In both Lae and Monrovia, there are few if any safe
houses, and neither city had well established child protective services.
This meant that people usually had no choice but to return to where
they were abused.

The establishment of access to safe termination of pregnancy is another challenge. Women and girls who are raped and become pregnant are twice as likely to have an abortion,[vi] and in places where abortion is legally restricted this can be extremely dangerous. In Liberia, we saw many pregnant teenage girls who said their pregnancies were the only reason they told anyone that they had been raped. In hopes of terminating the pregnancy, many had done terrible things to themselves—inserted sticks or lye into their vaginas, for example—or had paid someone else to do it for them. There was something in Liberia called an "RPG," as in rocket-propelled grenade: a combination of herbs and lye and chemicals that they would insert into themselves. Frequently these attempts would go horribly wrong, and the girls and women would come to us badly wounded or very ill, some with life-threatening injuries.

Incidents like these, which occur in numerous countries around the world, show how important it is that safe abortion services are made available. As we see repeatedly, the alternatives can be fatal.

As difficult as it can be to persuade victims of sexual violence to come for medical services, we know community outreach can work. After we let people know where to come for care in Lae, patients started arriving. We had billboards in town, we did radio shows, and made weekly visits to community markets and churches to spread the word that victims of sexual violence should come get treatment within 72 hours of the attack. The more outreach we did, the more women and girls came in within those crucial 72 hours. We knew this wasn't everyone, but it was a good start. Sexual violence must be acknowledged in a community for things to start to change. In 2012, the third year of MSF's program in Lae, after we'd conducted outreach and advocacy, we noticed an enormous change in how society talked about violence, including rape. More people in the community, in parliament, and the Ministry of Health acknowledged the problem and called for action.

However, a major barrier to expanding community engagement is the lack of existing data—numbers that can reinforce the demands for change. MSF can point to the numbers of patients treated at its projects in PNG, but there are no recent official numbers on the prevalence of sexual violence. Reporting methods in the country must change for the government to get a clear picture of the extent of sexual violence.

The issue extends beyond PNG: currently there is no reliable way to know how many women, men and children have suffered sexual violence around the world. The closest study we have is one published by the WHO in 2013 that looks at violence in general. It found that around 35 percent of all women "will experience either intimate partner or non-partner violence," which includes but is not limited to sexual violence.[vii] We lack a study that shows the scope of the problem of sexual violence, which makes it more difficult to press the international community, governments and communities to take action.

Changing systems and policies and reducing the stigma carried by victims of sexual violence requires time, resources, and political will. To start the process, treatment and support must be made available to anyone who needs it. And when care is available, people must know how to gain access to it. In Liberia, for instance, MSF's small, three-person medical and mental health team saw 150 victims of sexual violence per month due to our outreach activities. But we know that was just the tip of the iceberg.

You Are Not Alone
By Aerlyn Pfeil, Midwife, CPM, BSM

In 2013, I was working in Wardher, a town in Ethiopia's Somali region. One night, I woke up to hear a woman screaming, clearly in distress. Then I heard other voices, another woman yelling. I remember thinking it sounded like a woman was being raped and murdered. It was horrible.

There are many different armed factions fighting in this volatile, perpetually neglected region of the country. It's a place where women and girls are extremely vulnerable to rape and assault.

The sounds were coming from directly behind the walled MSF compound in the village. The MSF guard came to ask me if he could go see what was going on; by then, we had also heard gunfire. I was too worried that something would happen to him if he went, so I told him not to. Unless someone came to us to get help, we'd have to wait and see what happened the next day.

In the morning, we found out that a woman I knew, Hannah, had been attacked and that she and her children had been detained. I got permission to bring her some medication and to have a brief private conversation with her. After she was finally released, we talked more. She told me that she wanted me to share her story. A man who belonged to an armed group and lived not far from her hut had broken in and sexually assaulted her and her daughter. When they could, Hannah and her son fought back, eventually chasing the man out of their house. The man then fired his gun to alert other men from his group to come, but luckily no one did. The police came the following day and took Hannah and her children to jail.

Hannah's attacker turned up at our emergency room seeking treatment for his head injuries. (I was in the maternity ward and did not see him; to practice the MSF principle of neutrality in this instance would have been extremely difficult.) The assault on Hannah and her daughter was among the most disturbing events that occurred during my time working with MSF. With incidents like these, there was nothing I could do except to help the victims as best I could, giving them the best possible care. But this effort comes with huge challenges.

MSF supports several departments of the hospital in Wardher, offering antenatal care and maternity services, treatment for severe malnutrition, and pediatric care. It also runs the emergency room and the tuberculosis (TB) ward. The staff sees two to three victims of violence-related trauma every day—mostly people with wounds from gunshots, knives, burnings, or beatings, along with victims of sexual violence, most of whom are girls under the age of 18.

In 2013, the team treated 33 survivors of sexual violence and five others who the team suspected had been raped. The patient numbers alone give the deceptive impression that sexual violence is not a major issue in Wardher. But after conducting interviews with the community that year, the maternity team estimated that less than 10 percent of sexual violence survivors in the area sought care.

In Wardher, rape is defined as forced sex outside of marriage (rape between husband and wife is not acknowledged). Unmarried women and girls who are raped lose value as potential wives—they may even be forced to marry the perpetrator. These social dynamics make it extremely difficult for victims to seek care.

As in Hannah's case, husbands and fathers often migrate to other parts of Ethiopia or Somalia to find work and women and children are left alone. Children are frequently charged with tending livestock and collecting water by themselves. Many women and teenagers told us that armed men go house to house and ask the children if the father is home. If he is away, they will return to harass and rape the women.

One woman we met, Ruth, lived in a tiny hut with five small children whose father had not been around for months. "The men know I have no husband," she told me during a visit. "They come into my house in the evening and they drink all my water, all my tea, they eat all my food, and they can do whatever they want. I have no power."

Ruth had not been raped, but she said she would be eventually and she knew she would have no recourse. "What can I do?" she said. "These are the people who supply my water. These are the people who are supposed to protect me."

In Ethiopia as in numerous countries, it is difficult for women to come into a hospital and say, "I have been raped. Please help." In Wardher, doing so could be dangerous. Knowing we had to work with these realities, we concluded that the best way to reach women and provide them access to services for sexual violence was to go to them, in their homes and communities.

In 2014, during my second assignment in Wardher, our small sexual violence team initiated a form of private, home-based care for survivors of sexual violence. We went from house to house in town, giving health information talks. While speaking with groups of women, teenagers, men, and community elders about why they should vaccinate their children and why women should come to the hospital when they're in labor, we also talked about sexual violence.

Including the topic in a broader discussion about health made it more acceptable, less intrusive. This gave us more space to talk about the potential medical consequences of rape and the confidential services available at the hospital.

The talks allowed the team to gather a lot more information. We learned that the perpetrators women were most afraid of were "those with guns." They could be soldiers, the militia, rebels, or other armed groups; the women were hesitant to make a distinction. But it was clear that women were more comfortable coming to the hospital if they had been raped by a civilian as opposed to an armed man.

In recent years, three Ethiopian staff members in Wardher had travelled to Nairobi to receive MSF's international training on sexual violence. Those staff and I trained the other midwives and community health workers to identify signs and symptoms of sexual violence, and how to provide basic counseling. The training emphasized how to talk about sexual violence in one's own community, and we encouraged them to use the appropriate messages. They ended up writing a song in which they described the health consequences of sexual violence. For these Somali women, who don't speak about such things very often, it was a pretty powerful song.

Once we started to direct attention to the issue, we saw growing interest in it. Each week, we met with local groups, including traditional birth attendants, to get our message out and keep the conversation alive. More talking did not necessarily translate into more care, though. As of mid-2014, the number of victims coming in had not risen much. I am also a survivor of sexual violence and I didn't get medical treatment. I didn't seek legal recourse, and my life wouldn't have been at risk if I had. This is why I knew that we needed to be patient. I want to see organizations like MSF and national health systems make a difference for these women, but care providers have to commit to the process and understand that it will take a lot of time, training, and sensitivity. Everyone must examine their own discomfort with the subject of rape. The messages will need to be repeated constantly.

For an emergency medical organization like MSF, it can be difficult to prioritize a problem as hidden as sexual violence, especially when so many other issues need attention. It is just as easy for governments to overlook sexual violence. But the problem is there.

Another challenge that is not widely understood is the reoccurrence of trauma. Many of the staff who work in these programs have social and economic circumstances similar to our patients. The female staff I worked with in Wardher expressed the same fears of violence. They felt at risk. Victims of sexual violence may heal physically, but the pain will always be with them. If a female health worker is caring for victims of sexual violence, her own experience with sexual violence could surface, and she will need support.

Even staff who have not suffered from violence first-hand face the effects of suffering or trauma. Health care providers can do a better job of helping staff recognize their own sources of anxiety and distress, and then supporting them.

Lately, the situation with armed groups in Wardher has worsened, and the lot of women there has worsened along with it. As in all our programs, MSF cannot prevent violence. But our care providers must be creative to find ways to reach women. We still have a long way to go.

MSF began treating victims of sexual violence 15 years ago when the organization recognized how simple interventions such as prophylaxis for HIV and unwanted pregnancy could keep patients from suffering even more. The obstacles to providing treatment remain enormous. At MSF projects, teams focus on areas where they can make an impact: ensuring confidentiality, encouraging people to come early for treatment, and convincing patients to get follow-up care. MSF also advocates for and at times provides direct assistance to help governments recognize sexual violence as a medical emergency and improve treatment and reporting systems.

But among the most challenging aspects of responding to sexual violence is dealing with stigma and shame. They enable rape because they keep victims silent and afraid. In some cultures, the social rejection that follows rape has the potential to cripple victims for the rest of their lives. It is no wonder sexual violence remains a hidden problem.

As with so many other difficult challenges, governments, health authorities, MSF and other health care providers must commit to working against sexual violence by reaching out to victims in any setting. While MSF projects are likely to see only a fraction of the people who need treatment for sexual violence, we have also seen that in providing the care, and in talking about the issue again and again over time, more women, girls, men and boys will seek the care that they need.

[i] Outreach Programme on the Rwanda Genocide at the United Nations, "Background Information on Sexual Violence used as a Tool of War." Accessed December 2014. http://www.un.org/en/preventgenocide/rwanda/about/bgsexualviolence.shtml

[ii] Conflict Profile: Women's Media Center, "Bosnia, Women Under Siege Project." 2012. http://www.womenundersiegeproject.org/conflicts/profile/bosnia

[iii] U.N., "Ending Violence Against Women and Girls," United Nations' Resources for Speakers on Global Issues. Accessed December 2014. http://www.un.org/en/globalissues/briefingpapers/endviol/

[iv] Rachel Jewkes et al, "Gender Inequitable Masculinity and Sexual Entitlement in Rape Perpetration South Africa: Findings of a Cross-Sectional Study." PLoS ONE. December 28, 2011. http://www.plosone.org/article/info%3Adoi%2F10.1371%2Fjournal.pone.0029590

[v] Amnesty International, "Briefing to the UN Committee on the Elimination of Discrimination Against Women," p. 9. 2009. http://www2.ohchr.org/english/bodies/cedaw/docs/ngos/AI_PapuaNewGuinea46.pdf

[vi] WHO Fact Sheet, "Violence Against Women," updated November 2014. http://www.who.int/mediacentre/factsheets/fs239/en/Ibid.

[vii] Ibid.

STORIES FROM PATIENTS

Claudia, 17, Guatemala City, Guatemala

Claudia's Mother: "Claudia had told me before that some boys were bothering her and that she was afraid. She went to work one afternoon and then at 6 p.m. I received a phone call. They told me they had my daughter and that they were going to give her back to me some other day, that they were going to have fun with her.

[Several hours later] a neighbor called me and told me that she saw Claudia walking towards the house. She said Claudia was barefoot, her hair was a mess, she looked as if she were drugged. It was very difficult for us to go through those distressing moments, but thank God they gave her back to us alive.

We think this is somebody we know. We made a statement at the police station. Then we dropped the charges for the same reason, because we thought it was someone we know and he might learn about the statement and perhaps do more harm later on.

Nobody informed us about taking her to a doctor. A friend took us to find a hospital but the hospital was no longer where it used to be. We had no idea of what else to do. It never crossed my mind about her having a venereal disease or anything. I was so devastated that I couldn't think of anything else. We did get her to a hospital, but much later."

Claudia: "A friend of my mom's recommended the MSF clinic and said we could talk to a woman there. I got all the vaccines against infection and I was screened for HIV. I began with my therapy. It was a very long process. The hardest thing at the time was finding out I was pregnant.

We attended therapy every eight days, then we started to have appointments every 15 days. It helped a lot. With such a problem, you can't do it alone. You need to feel others' support. Because you really feel very lonely, very abandoned and often very despised because of what you've been through. And you feel that it only happened to you.

It was very hard and sometimes very bitter. But I have overcome a lot.

I think the government is not paying enough attention to sexual abuse because they're more focused on [deadly] violence. They should consider how to help people who've gone through this. It's often not reported and it's not fully understood. You don't hear much about it because people don't talk about it when in fact it's something that happens every day."

Aurelia, Mother of Three, Honduras

"I live in an outlying neighborhood between two very dangerous districts. *[After a girl was raped by intruders in her house]* our neighbors got together and made a team to watch the neighborhood. Then two sons of people in the team were killed. So, they decided to stop watching. Then the *"mareros"* [*members of the Mara Salvatrucha gang*] took over the neighborhood.

I was walking to work at 5 o'clock in the morning when a white sedan with tinted windows stopped next to me. They rolled down the window and pulled out a gun and told me to get in. I tried to keep walking and the car kept moving backwards. They said, 'get in or we shoot you.' A man got out and put me in the car. They put tape on my hands and mouth and told me if I screamed they'd kill me.

They took me to a hotel. They were getting high and then they undressed me, started stroking me, kissing me. I asked them not to hurt me. They put me on the bed and began to have sex with me. After one got up, I tried to get up, and they pushed me back on the bed. Then it was the turn of the other one. Afterwards I saw him going to the table where the gun was. I begged them, 'I have children, please don't kill me.' He said, 'I'm not asking you. Shut up.' He put the gun on my forehead. I felt like dying. I just closed my eyes and he said, 'If you speak, I'll find you anywhere and I'll kill you.'

I stayed there I don't know for how long. One of the hotel maids and another girl came in and they helped me get dressed. They talked to me but I couldn't say anything. I began to cry, calling for my family.

When I got home I was so angry and I didn't want to leave the house. I didn't receive any medical care at first. Later, when my family took me to go look at photographs to try to identify the men, someone told my mother about MSF.

We went to MSF and they gave me medication and tended to me and I started receiving counseling there. At first, I couldn't speak. I couldn't tell what had happened because I was terrified. There was a time when I thought of ceasing to exist. Thanks to the therapy, I have gotten better. I will continue with it until I really know I'm fine. I have to heal that memory so that it no longer mortifies me.

I stayed alive because there are other people who are killed. There are women who are raped and remain silent and don't seek help out of fear or shame. But we all know that [rape] is not something that we seek, but something they force on us against our will."

Karen, Mother of Four, Honduras

"My attacker was my own husband. I was working the night shift. I had been trying to stay away from him and he started following me.

One day in November my children asked me for permission to go to their aunt's place for the weekend and when they went, they left the door open. That is how he came in. When I arrived home, he was already there and I didn't realize it. I went to bed and that is when he attacked me. He waited until I fell asleep.

Afterwards I didn't do anything. Mostly out of fear or shame. What I did was lock myself in my house. I didn't look for any kind of help from anybody. I stood right there, stuck. It was three or four months before I went to the health center.

I didn't know about the need to go to a doctor within 72 hours. If I'd known, I would have gone. I didn't go until I couldn't bear my own burden or my own guilt anymore. I felt guilty, mainly because I thought, 'if maybe I had noticed [that he was in the house], it wouldn't had happened.' The day I came to the health center was a horrible day. I felt bad, I just cried. I felt worthless, like nobody. I was nothing.

Before, I didn't leave my house. I didn't take my children to school. I didn't check on how they were doing. I was fired from the place where I worked because I lost control in such a way that I couldn't work anymore. Before this happened, I used to interact with everybody. Now I stand aside. I used to have friends, but it's not like that anymore.

At the beginning, I had to come here on foot and that was very difficult, but I wanted to move forward. I wanted to get better, to overcome what had happened to me. I have moved forward thanks to the support of the doctors who treated me during those difficult times.

At first, I couldn't accept what I was bearing in my womb. I didn't want him. Nine months passed and I couldn't accept that I was bearing a child. I was scared. I was afraid of looking at him after he was born. But thanks to the help I received, I could overcome it. When I saw him, I felt love for the child.

I feel I just need to do my part and here I am, working hard on that. Because that's my best wish, having a job to support my children. They depend only on me. They get no other help.

The truth of the matter is that we can't live like that. It is painful. It's something that affects you psychologically, and it not only affects the person but the whole family. I feel it affected my children. Even though they don't know anything, it did affect them as well."

Three Migrants' Stories in Morocco

Marie, 30, left Cameroon for North Africa in trying to reach Europe. She was raped several times on her way to Morocco and in Tamanrasset, Algeria, she was taken by a network that trafficks in illegal migrants and was forced into prostitution. She managed to run away and return to Morocco, only to find she was pregnant. She delivered a baby boy in Rabat.

"Our journey is not the journey that others see. When you are alone, when you don't have anywhere to sleep or you don't know the country; you are exposed.

In Tamanrasset, they take the women, search them one by one, undress them and rob them, take their mobiles, their money, even their dresses. And if they like you, they have sex with you.

We stayed there, and then they tell you they want to help you, but then when the night comes, then they start the job on your body. They beat you. They do what they want. If you don't want to, they make you leave and the police come and take you.

I don't know if it was the second or third rape. I have to tell [my son] the truth. You can't hide it. It's a story that I will always tell, even if I go to Europe and one day I get married, I will always tell my story."

Beauty, 32, left Ivory Coast during the 2011 war there. She says her name was on a list of those supporting the wrong man for president. She witnessed members of her family being killed. Beauty left her child with her father, who was not politically marked, and set off for Europe. In Tamanrasset, Algeria, she said she was raped by two men.

"He covered my mouth with his hand and he raped me. Then the other one came and raped me. They did it again and again, two people taking turns. I was suffocating and lost consciousness. When I woke up I was all wet, they had thrown water on me. I couldn't speak. They dressed me and took me back to where they had caught me. They left me there."

When she was in Maghnia, near the Moroccan border, she was raped again. She was tricked by a seemingly friendly woman who brought her with some friends to a house. "After getting there, they locked the door, they gave me a blanket, and I thought that maybe they are kind. But that night they started raping me."

Beauty became infected with HIV and tuberculosis. She received medical and psychological care from MSF in Rabat, Morocco. She hopes she will recover from TB and get healthy again.

"In my country if you have HIV you are isolated, you are marginalized. You have become the black beast. If I was not killed in my country, or on the way here, and if this disease has not killed me, it is because God has something in store for me and wants me alive."

Aimee was raped by armed men during the 2011 war in Ivory Coast. She left and worked for a year at a restaurant in Mali, which was also threatened by war. She decided to join a group of people heading for Europe. During the journey, the man who had organized it took her as his "wife."

When they arrived in Algeria, she was sold to the man's friends. "He said, 'She is my companion, I have bought her. You can do with her whatever you want.'"

Aimee was then forced into a human smuggling network. She was sexually exploited and forced to work as a slave.

"I was there six months. The work we were forced to do was very hard. We had to fill sacks with sand and carry them, take very big stones and drag them. It was very difficult, but if you failed to do it, you weren't given food. And if you refused, they raped you again."

Aimee made it out and went to Rabat, Morocco. Many African women are forced into prostitution in Rabat, but she is not going to be one, she says. Her dream is to get to Europe and start a chain of beauty salons.

The Evolution Of Preventing Mother-To-Child Transmission Of HIV

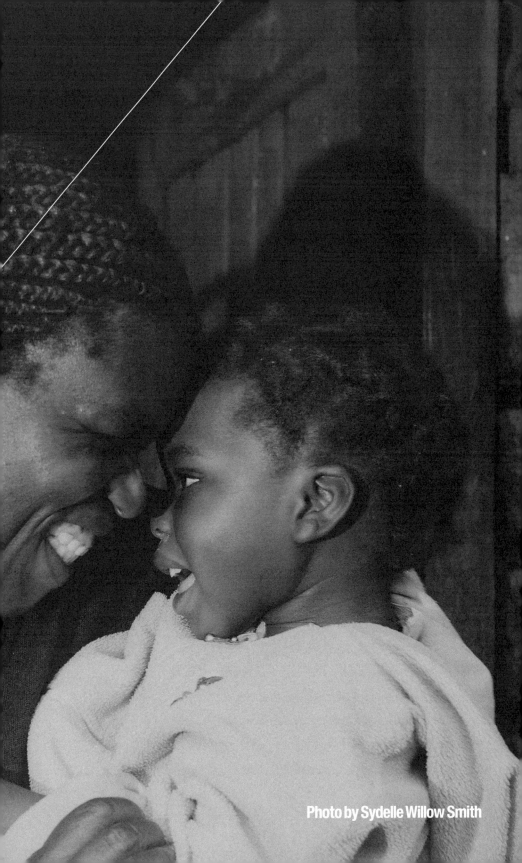

Photo by Sydelle Willow Smith

Chapter 6
The Evolution of Preventing Mother-to-Child Transmission of HIV

Better Treatment, Same Challenges
By Dr. Helen Bygrave, MBBS, MA, MRCP, MRCGP

One afternoon in 2006, Julia, 24, somehow found her way to my clinic room in the hospital in Lagos, Nigeria, where MSF was working. She was extremely weak—breathless, dizzy, and coughing. She was also 22 weeks pregnant and alone: her husband had died a month earlier. She had a five-year-old son, but her last two babies had died.

Given Julia's condition, just getting to the clinic room had been an act of sheer determination. For the past two months, she had been coughing badly and displaying several other symptoms typical of tuberculosis (TB) as well. This was not surprising: people living with HIV without treatment, whose immune systems are deteriorating, are particularly susceptible to opportunistic diseases like TB. Julia was also anemic. After she had learned that she'd tested positive for HIV, the hospital's antenatal care staff had directed her to MSF's small HIV clinic in the same building.

We admitted her for a short stay at the hospital to give her a blood transfusion and started her on TB treatment. A few weeks later, we started her on antiretroviral therapy (ART) for HIV. Antiretrovirals had only recently become available in Nigeria, and we could finally provide something beyond treatment for opportunistic diseases and palliative care, which previously had been all we were able to offer. ART had come to be known as the Lazarus treatment because it extended the lives of people carrying the virus. What's more, it was also proving very effective in preventing mother-to-child transmission (PMTCT) of HIV from pregnant women, like Julia, to their unborn children. Without ART, the mother-to-child transmission rate can be as high as 40 percent. With ART, it can be reduced to less than 5 percent.[i]

Julia improved quickly. A colleague was in charge of her care, so after those initial visits, I didn't see her again for five months, until she called out my name in the hospital corridor. She looked so much healthier that I almost didn't recognize her. And she had a little three-month-old baby on her back who, much to my relief, had tested negative for HIV.

———————————

Around the world, HIV affects men and women alike. But in many of the places where MSF works, women are more at risk and more women suffer from the disease. In sub-Saharan Africa, for example, 60 percent of people living with the virus are female. On top of the numerous medical and social challenges women must contend with, they must also worry about transmitting HIV to their unborn babies and breastfeeding infants.

The international community has in recent years made significant progress in PMTCT treatment and strategies. According to the World Health Organization, 900,000 women worldwide received PMTCT in 2012 and coverage for the whole of Africa grew from 13 percent in 2005 to 59 percent in 2011.

At MSF projects, staff provided PMTCT to 18,489 women in 2013. Currently, MSF treats 341,600 women, men, and children living with HIV in more than 20 countries.

There is still a long way to go. The WHO also estimates that only 64 percent of the women who need these services in 21 "priority" African countries are actually getting them, and in Southeast Asia, only 16 percent of pregnant women with HIV are receiving PMTCT.[ii] This shortfall in coverage means that in 2013 some 700 children were newly infected with HIV every day,[iii] roughly 90 percent of them in sub-Saharan Africa.[iv]

In Nigeria, six years after Julia got lifesaving treatment for her and her baby, only 17 percent of pregnant women had access to PMTCT.[v] The message is clear: for every success story like Julia's, there are many more women who do not get the care they need.

MSF, which began working with people living with HIV in the 1990s, has tried to adapt its programs to extend the reach of HIV care in general and PMTCT care in particular to as many people as possible. One way has been by decentralizing our HIV projects, allowing patients to start treatment at primary care clinics close to where they live rather than requiring them to travel to the nearest hospital, which might be days away. This entails shifting certain tasks from doctors to nurses who are specially trained to initiate ART.

MSF has also integrated maternity care and counseling into many of its HIV projects and PMTCT into many of its maternity projects. A pregnant woman who tests positive for HIV can avail herself of all the services she needs, for her health and to protect her baby, in a single visit, often from a single nurse. Where possible, staff also offer both HIV and TB care under the same roof.

Teams are trying to take advantage of improved treatment strategies, as well. The number of a patient's CD4 cells (cells that help activate the immune system when they detect a virus or bacteria) has long been used to determine when a patient needs to receive ART. Until 2013, most PMTCT programs only gave ART to pregnant women whose CD4 counts showed that their immune system was drastically weakened and they needed treatment immediately for their own health.

Pregnant women whose CD4 counts were still high would get a prophylactic medicine called AZT and after they gave birth, their babies were given an ART syrup until they finished breastfeeding. This practice, called Option A, is still used in a number of countries. But in places where the shortage of high quality laboratory services and trained medical personnel mean many women can't even find out what their CD4 count is, many go without the care they need.

A newer alternative, Option B+, is gaining greater acceptance. It was recommended by the WHO as the best course of treatment for pregnant women in 2013. Option B+ was devised in Malawi, a country with limited access to CD4 lab testing. Designed to simplify and broaden PMTCT services, it calls for putting all pregnant women who test positive for HIV on an ART regimen right away, regardless of their CD4 count, and for keeping them on ART for the rest of their lives.

There are several potential advantages to the B+ approach. It is easier for the mother to take a tablet once a day than trying to get a young baby to take a syrup every day, as they must with Option A. What's more, if the mother remains in treatment, any future pregnancy is protected as long as the level of HIV in her blood remains low. The ART also provides health benefits for the mother herself. And since we now know that effective ART can render the amount of the virus in someone's blood and sexual secretions to be almost undetectable, it makes it that much more difficult to transmit HIV to one's spouse, partner—or baby during pregnancy and breastfeeding.

MSF is unable to guarantee lifelong ART in all of its PMTCT projects. Where national governments have not instituted a consistent system of care for HIV patients, those initiated on antiretroviral treatment have nowhere to go after PMTCT with MSF is complete. Most often the developing countries with the highest rates of HIV are the only ones that have established such a system, so MSF is limited to using Option B+ in countries with a high prevalence of the disease. Malawi, Swaziland, Zimbabwe and Lesotho are four examples, and in each, Option B+ is also part of the national treatment protocol.

Option B+ is extremely promising, but it is not a cure-all and it cannot end mother-to-child transmission by itself. Over the years, I have met women who have refused to start treatment—or defaulted on it once they began—because they were financially and socially dependent on their partners and feared that disclosing their HIV status would have disastrous consequences. Some have, amazingly, overcome these barriers, but others have not, and have suffered the inevitable outcome.

For those who are able to reach our treatment facilities, we have to make sure that we take into account the patient and the realities of her life. As Julia and many others have shown, women with HIV still have a great deal to live for.

Whatever It Takes, We Should Do
By Pamela A. Onango, RN, Midwife

In 2014, when I was working in Agok, South Sudan, I had a displaced, pregnant 26-year-old patient named Amal. She had come for antenatal care, which includes testing for HIV. She was very receptive to the health information, the explanation of what HIV is, and how it is treated. She was cooperative during the testing, too. But when I presented her with the results of her HIV test and told her that she had tested positive for the disease, she said, "No, it is not mine."

There were only the two of us in the consultation room. I had clearly drawn and tested her blood. I told her that yes, her result was positive for HIV, but she still would not accept it.

We decided to give her some time to think about it. In this project, we track all our patients. If someone does not come for follow-up, we reach out to them and ask them to come back, and we kept reaching out to her. She kept denying that she was HIV positive. She kept insisting that she couldn't be sick, she couldn't have the disease. We kept trying to convince her to get PMTCT treatment—if not for her own sake, than for the sake of her baby. But we were not successful.

Amal delivered at home, without having had any PMTCT care. We asked her to come for postnatal care where she would receive incentives like a mosquito net, a luxury in a camp in Agok. We still could have given the baby medication and Amal would not have had to take anything herself if she did not want to. But that would have been admitting she was sick and she could not do that.

It was very sad for us, for her baby, and for her. The baby could become symptomatic in the first few years of his or her life and could die;

Amal, too, could die as a result of her infection.

Testing is usually not the challenge; the challenge comes when we have the results. Every patient needs to understand what it means to have HIV and be on antiretroviral treatment. Many will grasp this only after extensive counseling, which takes time, because it's not always easy for people to accept the new reality and adjust to its ramifications for them and their families. Perhaps additional counseling could have helped Amal realize what needed to be done for her and her baby. A community better informed about HIV and treatment options would have helped as well.

I've worked in places with very high HIV prevalence rates, like Swaziland, where in 2012 more than a quarter of the general population was living with HIV, and where surveys conducted two years earlier had found that 41 percent of pregnant women were as well.[vi] The numbers are staggering, but many people in the country understand what HIV is and what can be done about it. In contrast, South Sudan's prevalence rate was estimated at 2.3 percent in 2013.[vii] Far fewer people were living with the virus, but also far fewer who knew what it was.

In both situations, there are opportunities to provide effective PMTCT. When there is already some understanding of what HIV is, it is easier to counsel mothers, to make them understand that there is treatment available, and advise them how to live a healthy life and protect their babies. I have seen mothers go to incredible lengths to protect their children, but there are many obstacles to proper care, including the stigma that still attends the disease.

In a country like South Sudan, there is a great opportunity to give people the right information about the disease and the treatment for it. But with no foundation of understanding and acceptance in the community, and no political willingness to deal with HIV at the policy level, misinformation spreads and people struggle to accept HIV and the importance of starting ART. I've seen community leaders say, "I have heard about HIV, but we don't have that in this country." It's not so different from Amal's refusal to accept her status.

Sometimes fears surround the medication; people worry that it is toxic or will affect one's features so that others will recognize that they have HIV. (This relates to old treatments that disfigured the face and muscles. With the newer regimens this does not happen.) MSF projects, therefore, stress community outreach and education. During the daily general health talks we give at MSF hospitals, our staff try to educate all patients about HIV. We also hire and train community health workers to visit people in their homes and in public places to raise awareness about HIV.

In Swaziland, a patient named Elizabeth came to us from outside the Nhlangano region. She was open about her status and, having already been through a PMTCT program elsewhere, she knew all about HIV treatment. Her CD4 count was still high, but she came to us during her second pregnancy because she wanted lifelong ART and had heard that MSF was running a pilot project in Nhlangano using Option B+. "I want to remain the way I am now and I am told that when you take this treatment you will not be sick with other diseases," she said. "And, one thing I am certain of is this will not be the last time I am pregnant."

Though she lived far away, Elizabeth stayed near the hospital to get treatment until she delivered. After that she was transferred back to her health zone and continued treatment. Her understanding of the disease and her determination to live to the fullest pushed her to seek out a treatment strategy that worked for her and her children. We also asked her to bring her husband for testing. They hadn't been married long and she hadn't told him she had HIV. As it happened, he had it, too, and he had been on ART for years.

This was a good outcome, leading to a better understanding among partners who learned the other was dealing with more than they would have imagined. Research has shown that a woman who has told her partner about her status is more likely to come for follow-up care. But in many cases, it does not go so smoothly. Many women are scared to tell their husbands they have HIV, and many husbands refuse to get testing or treatment for themselves or to take steps necessary—including using condoms—to protect their spouses, and thus their children, from HIV.

An intransigent or willfully ignorant partner can be a major obstacle for both treatment and prevention. I have had numerous patients tell me that they must "get consent" from the husband before making any decisions about starting ART. Sometimes I want to say, "Why are you asking your husband for permission to live?" Either they truly are not allowed to make these decisions or they are making an excuse to avoid a decision. In either case they clearly feel they lack the power to make it and that is a very big challenge.

Women need their partners' support, but men are not customarily involved in PMTCT. Men have pointed out to me that the name PMTCT includes the word mother but not father. "How are we involved in this?" they say. "If the mother wants the program, let the mother handle the program with the baby." They also tend to see the maternity department and antenatal care area as women's or children's places, so they don't think they should come in to be tested with their partner.

MSF is trying to change some male attitudes towards HIV and testing prevalence in places where we work. It's not so much a social issue for us as a medical one, a recognition that certain behaviors have profound public health consequences—especially for women and children. Right now in Gutu, Zimbabwe, for example, MSF teams are keeping the clinic open at night, when men seem to be more willing to come in, and getting patients who test positive on treatment immediately. So far, 70 percent of those tested have been men.

We also need to encourage men to be more involved in PMTCT. I wonder if we should call it Prevention of Parent-to-Child Transmission, to make it more inclusive. We should do whatever it takes to remove these challenges and get more women (and men) in treatment.

A Shift in Thinking and Treating
By Joanne Cyr, Psy.D.

Sylvia came into our counseling room at Arua Regional Referral Hospital in Uganda one afternoon, carrying her three-month-old baby. She had previously tested positive for HIV and was on ART to prevent her from transmitting the virus to her child, according to the PMTCT Option A approach. She had been bottle-feeding the child with something—cow's milk, perhaps. In this area of scarce food, most women would not have had access to alternatives to breast milk.

This was in 2011 and the health staff were strongly encouraging women, including those living with HIV, to breastfeed their babies exclusively. Breastfeeding provides a child with rich protective immunoglobulins and nutrients that they will not get from any other source. It's not always obvious to young mothers, though, and they need support and guidance. It was all the more distressing when the health ministry nurse and midwives at the hospital openly disparaged Sylvia's decision to not breastfeed.

In response, I met with Sylvia and introduced her to the "peer mothers," a group of three women MSF had hired and trained as peer counselors. They were members of our PMTCT Mothers Support Group and had already been through the PMTCT program. MSF uses "expert patients" like these women in many different projects. They are able to help guide women like Sylvia through the same difficult journey they had made.

In Arua, the peer mothers worked closely with the patients from diagnosis to delivery and after. Two peer mothers taught daily health education at the hospital and offered one-on-one support. Another, Jane, was in the antenatal room where the ministry of health staff offered routine HIV testing. She would speak with women who were being tested and spent extra time with those who tested positive. She would also offer to accompany them to the PMTCT clinic for education and enrollment.

The peer mothers told Sylvia how they had breastfed their own babies, who were still free of HIV. In talking with her further, however, Jane discovered that Sylvia was deeply afraid that she might infect her baby through breastfeeding, even if she followed every guideline we gave her. Jane also learned that Sylvia was an educated woman who knew a lot about HIV and that she could afford to buy formula. In the end, the peer mothers helped Sylvia make an informed choice to bottle-feed her baby with formula safely, without any other foods that could put the child at risk. Peer mothers are able to use their own experience and take into account mothers' personal fears and history. They add a much needed personal element to a clinical setting.

At nine months old, Sylvia's baby tested negative for HIV. I helped the doctor deliver the news, and Sylvia expressed gratitude to the entire team for their support.

In 2013, when MSF was launching a PMTCT Option B+ pilot program in Nhlangano, Swaziland, I met Trinity, an exceptionally skillful peer counselor living with HIV who was trained by the South African peer support organization Mother-to-Mother. She helped us refine our patient information messages for the launch and helped counsel mothers in the program. I was lucky enough to see her in action one day.

The nursing staff had just diagnosed as HIV-positive a patient who was six months pregnant and sitting with her two-year-old on her lap. Trinity immediately joined her and delivered just the right amount of information, reassurance, and recommendations. I suggested that she accompany the mother to the nearby health center to have an antenatal care exam and get a prescription for antiretrovirals, and she agreed.

Trinity helped the woman formulate a plan to disclose her status first to her sister-in-law, and then to her partner. Her partner agreed to come in for testing, along with the two-year-old. He tested positive; the toddler was negative. Trinity counseled the couple together and got them started on taking lifelong ART.

Even with peer mothers' involvement, programs offering integrated HIV and maternity care face significant challenges, much of them related to limited human resources. Patients do not always get the confidential space they need in this environment, although privacy and confidentiality are an essential part of PMTCT. I've even seen women being tested for HIV in front of other women in the waiting room. Men who come in with their partners will usually refuse to get tested in this situation.

What's more, women often do not get proper counseling. In my training sessions I've asked for feedback from staff working in these projects and have been told that proper counseling takes too long when they have 30 other women who need testing and counseling as well. We talk about this a lot, and the point I try to drive home is that if you counsel a woman properly, she will be more of an agent in her own health care over the long term—she can make informed decisions and stick with the decision she makes. She can also develop skills for discussing health issues with her partner.

This is the essence of patient-centered care, but it's an approach that takes time to instill. Staff in HIV programs must follow national or other guidelines that are by necessity very regimented and clear-cut. There is not a lot of room for making individual assessments. Asking people to use their clinical or personal judgment, and to make decisions based on the needs of the individual patients involves asking them to adapt. It's a big shift, but it's a necessary one. A health worker has to be able to take in a patient and her personal circumstances regarding her family and community, her strengths, vulnerabilities and particular challenges, and help her accordingly.

Treatment for HIV has come a very long way in the last two decades, but the fight is not over. The availability of affordable generic antiretrovirals in developing countries since the 2000s has saved countless lives. Prevention of the transmission of the disease from mother to child has also taken leaps forward, especially with the advent of Option B+. But even today, many people who need ART are not receiving it, and Option B+ needs to be available in more countries, including those that do not have high rates of HIV, to better protect the next generation and their mothers.

A major battle must be won against the stigma that still surrounds

HIV, which prevents women, pregnant or otherwise, from getting treatment. The stigma prevents men from supporting or even allowing their partners to gain access to treatment (and keeps men from getting tested and started on treatment). More governments and communities need to take the lead in combating misinformation and stigma around HIV. Health care providers must engage men as much as possible in PMTCT, to strengthen their support.

Finally, peer mothers or expert patients are invaluable in PMTCT programs for the empathetic individual counseling they provide, among other reasons. They should be closely involved in care every step of the way. But given the sensitivity around HIV, staff members providing clinical care must also take into account individual needs, even if they feel overwhelmed by their workload. Women need discreet, supportive and responsive care. This is another challenge that will take time and a lot of reinforcement, but it must be done to get results.

In many instances, a woman who tests positive for HIV will immediately ask, "Am I going to live?" The very next question is often, "Can I raise a family?" Health care staff have to be ready to help every woman through these questions and those that follow. Her treatment, her future, and the futures of her children depend on it.

[i] WHO, "Mother-to-child transmission of HIV." http://www.who.int/hiv/topics/mtct/en/
[ii] UNICEF, "The First Decade of Life." Updated 2013; http://www.unicef.org/aids/index_firstdecade.html
[iii] UNAIDS, Epi Slides, p. 20. http://www.unaids.org/sites/default/files/media_asset/01_Epi_slides_2014July.pdf
[iv] UNICEF, "Towards an AIDS-Free Generation-Children and AIDS Stocktaking Report." 2013, p. 2. http://data.unicef.org/corecode/uploads/document6/uploaded_pdfs/corecode/str6_full_report_29-11-2013_78.pdf
[v] WHO, "Global Update on HIV Treatment: Results, Impact and Opportunities." 2013; http://www.who.int/hiv/pub/progressreports/update2013/en/
[vi] UNAIDS, "Swaziland Country Report on Monitoring the Political Declaration on HIV and AIDS." March 2012. http://www.unaids.org/sites/default/files/en/dataanalysis/knowyourresponse/countryprogressreports/2012countries/ce_SZ_Narrative_Report[1].pdf
[vii] South Sudan HIV/AIDS Commission, UNAIDS, "Global AIDS Response Progress Report, Country: South Sudan." March 2014. http://www.unaids.org/sites/default/files/country/documents/SSD_narrative_report_2014.pdf

STORIES FROM PATIENTS AND STAFF

Alice, 33, Kibera, Kenya

"I have two kids and I am eight months pregnant. The first time I came to MSF, I was sick and pregnant with my second child. I came to get antenatal care and I was referred to get tested. I tested HIV-positive.

I was very afraid when I was told, but there was good counseling and it helped a lot. I accepted my status and started treatment immediately. My first-born is HIV-positive. For my second pregnancy, I really adhered to my treatment. I made sure I had good nutrition and I went to the hospital for delivery. I made sure I breastfed her without feeding her anything else. When she was tested, she was HIV-negative.

In Kibera [a poor neighborhood in Nairobi], our parents really don't give us information about sex, which puts us at higher risk for getting infected. I'm a health educator now and I use my own experience to teach people. When I meet teenage girls, I always talk to them about prevention. I even go as far as demonstrating to them how to use a condom more effectively. It's not a matter of abstinence most of the time. If they learn prevention with a condom, that's more important.

I learned I was HIV-positive in 2007. People didn't have information about HIV then. I see a great change now; the stigma has been reduced and I've been accepted in the community. Now I'm very comfortable telling people I am HIV-positive. Nevertheless, people still become afraid when they find out; they stigmatize you. So it's difficult.

As a woman, disclosing your status to your husband is difficult. Sometimes it brings more violence in the house, which increases the risk of infection. Women often don't have the power to negotiate with their husbands.

I met my current husband in a support group. He knew my status and I knew his. I'm very happy right now. At first I could not even talk of my HIV status. But now I've been empowered. I have information and I take the initiative to empower women in the rural areas because there are no organizations there. That's my personal initiative. They even come to me at home if they have any concerns. I want to help people and try to reduce HIV infection, especially among those who are not getting the information.

Since MSF has been here there has been an improvement. It is not as before, when we used to have to walk for long distances seeking health care. However, there is no employment here so you gather grain and find small game, and sometimes it is not enough to raise my kids and pay the rent. These are real challenges for me."

Mary, in Myanmar

"I went to the doctor because I was suffering from enlarged lymph nodes on my neck. The hospital was screening everyone for HIV and that is how I found out I was HIV-positive. When I got my results I was shocked. I went home and stayed there. I did not go out.

Eventually I learned about a local NGO and they gave me information about MSF. That is how I came to this clinic. The MSF staff asked me to bring my partner to the clinic to get the HIV test as well. My husband tested positive, too. His CD4 count was very low—180.

Eight months later I found out I was pregnant. I didn't get out of bed. I stopped eating and lost weight. I was so anxious and worried about my baby. But I talked with my husband and we went together to the MSF clinic to find out what could be done. We got counseling and talked to the doctors. I got information on how to reduce the risk of transmission to the baby and that helped me calm down. If I had not gotten this information, I know I would have stayed home and my child would have gotten infected with HIV.

I have not disclosed my status to my family, only my husband. I think they would discriminate against me. I see a lot of discrimination in my community. If someone has HIV, no one visits that house. A girl with HIV died recently and no one went and helped with her funeral.

I don't know if she did not get treatment because she didn't have any information or because she blamed herself and was in denial. It could have been either. It takes me three hours to reach the clinic every time I come. I take a boat across the river, then a bus, to get here. But other patients have to come from even farther away. My only concern is for how long MSF will be able to provide me with antiretrovirals."

Pamela, 14, Malawi

"I am 14 years old and I have one child, a son. I went for an antenatal check-up at the health center. They tested me and told me I am HIV-positive, the virus that causes AIDS. They told me they were going to give me medication, but since I am a minor I had to go get my parents. I asked my parents to go with me to the health center and they refused, so I asked my elder sister. She's the one who allowed me to start my antiretroviral therapy.

My mother said that since she was not there when I got HIV, it should not affect her. I felt bad. I felt this is not like my mother. It affected me. It really hurt. Sometimes the family wouldn't give me food to eat. Sometimes I had to sleep outside the house.

My mother would take the flour bucket and hide it so I could not eat at all. My sister supported me the way I needed, but the rest of the family did not help me at all. My mother and I are still not on very good terms.

As of now, my son is HIV-negative. I thank God for the help I receive every time I go to the PMTCT program. I think other girls can benefit from the counseling as I did, if they are open enough to go to the health facility to get it.

What I'm planning for the future is to get my son tested again at 24 months. When I confirm it's negative, I will look for work, even for housework. What I need is money to support my son."

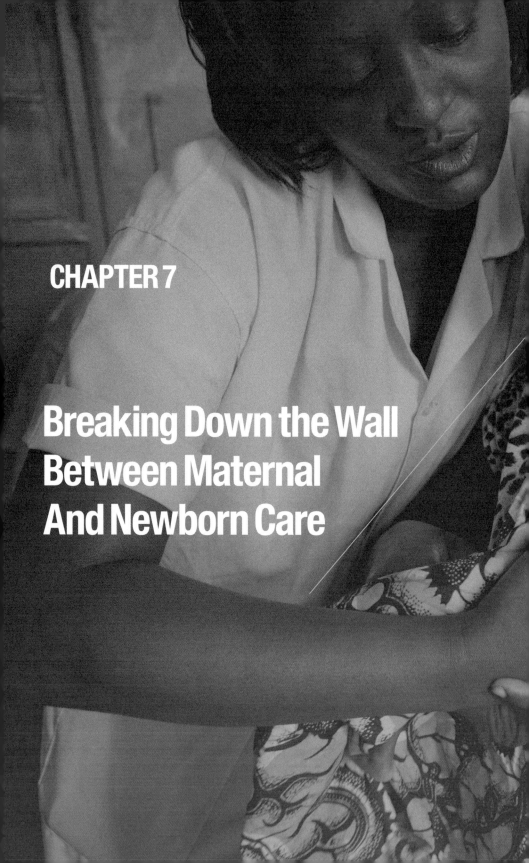

CHAPTER 7

Breaking Down the Wall Between Maternal And Newborn Care

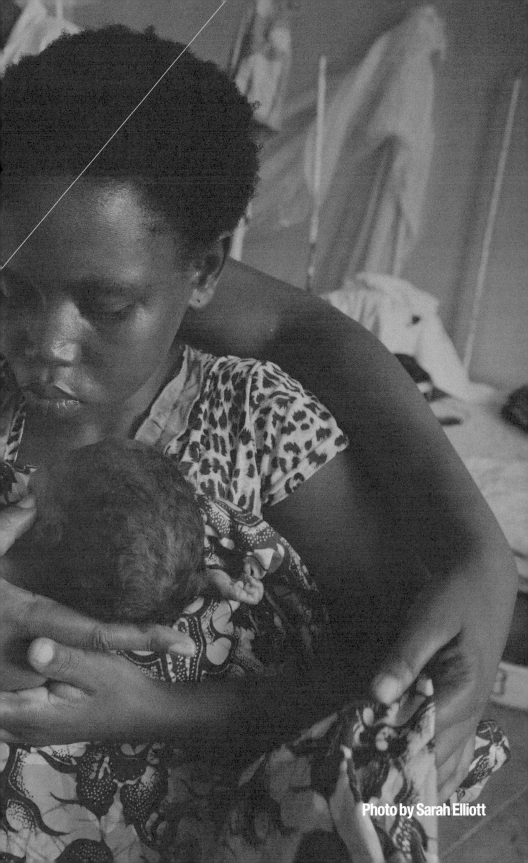

Photo by Sarah Elliott

Chapter 7
Breaking Down the Wall Between Maternal and Newborn Care

By Kristin Hooper, RN, BSN,
with Dr. Nicolas Peyraud, MD

One day in 2013, Mary Abuk, a beautiful 19-year-old, delivered triplets about 12 weeks prematurely in the MSF-supported hospital in Aweil, South Sudan. Two of the babies were stillborn, but one survived, a tiny little boy. He weighed only 900 grams (less than two pounds), and our staff set about doing everything they could to save him.

This child needed swift and effective care, something too often unavailable for mothers like Mary Abuk. Aweil sits in a region where medical care for newborns and their mothers—or medical care of any kind—has long been in short supply.

Over time, many parents have grown resigned to losing children in the earliest stages of their lives. They are no less heartbroken, but many are reluctant to invest any hope in the possibility that a baby as underweight and frail as Mary Abuk's son would make it through the day.

Mary Abuk, however, was determined to fight for her tiny son. She named him Deng Deng—"deng" means rain in the Dinka language—and she would stay with him in the hospital for the next two months.

MSF offers reproductive care in 159 projects worldwide. In 2013, MSF teams delivered 182,234 babies.

In those early hours and days, the staff provided Deng Deng with all the standard elements of newborn care, keeping him in a warm room and making sure that Mary fed him every two to three hours with formula that we provided. The staff also administered IV fluids and antibiotics throughout the week.

With support from her own mother and guidance from the MSF team, Mary Abuk also performed "kangaroo care" for Deng Deng: the staff showed her how to wrap the baby close her chest, creating skin-to-skin contact that can help stabilize a baby's temperature, encourage lactation in the mother, and enhance bonding between mother and child. She cleaned him and the linens that touched him every day. When she needed a rest, her mother would take over.

It wasn't an easy process. Deng Deng, like all newborns, was highly susceptible to infections because, while he was equipped with antibodies from his mother, his own immune system was not yet developed enough to fend off infectious threats. And the smaller and weaker a baby is, the harder it is for their body to build up immunity.

Over the next two months, Deng Deng's health followed a pattern. He would get sick, then get better, then get sick again before recovering once more. Mary Abuk's spirits rose and fell with his condition. She would be overjoyed that he was doing well, then devastated because she was sure he was going to die.

Deng Deng permanently lost his sight during this period, the sort of complication that is not uncommon to prematurely born babies fighting for their lives. But in the end, he put on weight. He grew. He got stronger. Four months after he was born, Mary Abuk brought him in for a check-up, and where we once saw a tiny baby on the brink of death, we now saw a healthy little boy.

It was heartening for our whole team. Beyond that, though, it was a good example of what can be done in an under-resourced country to keep a sick newborn alive when staff know what to do and they work together with the mother to do it.

There are many babies like Deng Deng who never get the chance to survive because they and their mothers have no access to proper care. It might be due to a region's history of war or its lack of development. It might be that the import of newborn and maternal care is not well understood by the community or by some health workers. It might be some other factor.

Whatever the reasons, the lack of adequate newborn care in developing countries is a problem the international community has only recently begun to address in a serious way. While there has been an overall improvement in mortality of children under five—the number of child deaths dropped by about half between 1990 and 2013, according to a UN/World Bank report—other measurements of infant and neonatal death have not improved nearly as dramatically. In 1990, newborn deaths accounted for 37 percent of all under-five child deaths; in 2013, they accounted for 44 percent.[i]

Of the 6.6 million children under five years who died in 2012, more than 2.9 million died within 28 days of birth.[ii]

In 2000, the UN laid out its Millennium Development Goal 4: to reduce the mortality rate of children under five by two-thirds by 2015. As of early 2015, this goal had not yet been reached, and if more attention isn't paid to providing prompt and effective medical care for newborns, it may never be.[iii]

A child's health is most at risk in the first 28 days of life, the neonatal period. Put simply, all babies should receive basic newborn care. And neonatal care should be integrated with maternal care, meaning the staff treating mothers should be able to treat their newborns as well.

The health of the mother and the child are inextricably linked: the sort of care that most benefits newborns involves the mothers, and it should be sought out and offered before, during, and after the birth of the child. It may not require cutting-edge technology, but it does require diligence, attention, and skilled attendants.

It also requires an understanding that obstetric, antenatal, and postnatal care are not separate processes, but interconnected, all part of the effort to assist a mother through the birth process and protect her newborn from the threats a baby will inherently face upon entry into the world.

As the story of Mary Abuk and Deng Deng shows, there are certain steps and procedures that can save lives, even in places where resources are minimal. The majority of newborn deaths can in fact be prevented without sophisticated equipment or complex protocols. This is what MSF is trying to focus on.

When a mother gives birth in an MSF facility, the midwife or nurse examines the baby and advises the mother to stay for monitoring of both her and her baby. Ideally, they would stay for the baby's first 24 hours of life, though that often does not happen. With pre-term babies like Deng Deng (and full-term but underweight babies) the need to remain at the facility is crucial. These babies are at higher risk of dying in the first days of life, and the staff need to keep a close watch for the most common killers: asphyxia and sepsis (an invasive, usually bacterial infection), and complications from prematurity.

For babies born outside of an MSF facility in an unhygienic environment, staff also look for tetanus, a disease caused by exposure to a deadly bacteria that is particularly dangerous for newborns. This is also a time when staff can provide counseling, treatment, and vaccinations that a mother may have missed if she did not receive antenatal care (ANC).

After birth and for the following days and weeks, MSF provides postnatal care, or PNC. In the best case, a mother will come in with her baby at least twice in the first six weeks for check-ups and necessary vaccinations and treatments [See Chapter 2: Maternal Health Before and After Childbirth].

Knowing the steps we have to take for newborns and their mothers is one thing. Implementing them in some of the places where we work is something else. When you look at the contexts in which many newborns die, you can see that this does not happen in a vacuum, nor is it because of mothers' indifference.

Deng Deng, for instance, was born into one of the world's most challenging environments for newborns. His mother is part of a generation of men and women who grew up well before South Sudan was a country, during the protracted, bloody conflict between the Sudanese government and the Sudanese Peoples' Liberation Movement. The civil war lasted for two decades, and by the time the two sides agreed to a truce in 2005, it had killed a million and a half people, displaced four million more, and crippled the development of education and public health systems throughout the South.

Many of the women who came to the MSF hospital in Aweil told me that they had lost or been separated from their parents and other relatives during the civil war. Many were married very young and moved away from their families. So not only were there very few medical facilities or trained staff available in the area, but they had not benefitted from the transmission of knowledge about pregnancy and birth that their mothers would have possessed, given their own experiences.

As such, there were many misconceptions among women from the area, some of which were potentially dangerous. In Aweil and elsewhere in South Sudan, this knowledge vacuum is an often overlooked consequence of the civil war. (Our staff also sees the same dynamics at play in other countries with the highest neonatal mortality rates.)

MSF began neonatal care activities in Aweil hospital in 2008. Two years later, in response to the high rates of neonatal mortality in the area, the team created a separate neonatal care unit. It took some time to get everything working as it should in order to provide consistent, quality care.

Staffing was a particular difficulty, again due to the tolls of the civil war. Finding qualified health staff in a place where a whole generation was barely able to go to school continues to be an issue, but our teams were able to find people who could be taught what they needed to know. It's not only the local staff who need to be readied to work in this environment, though. Foreign-born midwives and OBGYNs must also be briefed on the scope and nature of their responsibilities in the field, which often go far beyond what they'd be doing at home.

The numbers in Aweil show what's possible when integrated maternal and neonatal protocols are combined with dedicated staff training. From 2011 to 2014, neonatal mortality inside the hospital dropped from 18.9 percent to 11.1 percent, while deliveries rose from 292 per month to 423 during the same period.

The progress does not lessen the challenges, however. The staff sees this every day.

One morning, a young woman I'll call Sarah came in with four-day-old twins, a boy and a girl she had delivered at home. They were low birth weight babies likely born several weeks premature, and she was struggling to find the time to give them the attention they needed because she had other children at home who also needed tending to. She nonetheless had brought them into the hospital when they started to look sickly.

It was too late for the little boy, who died soon after his mother arrived. The little girl was febrile, malnourished, and was having trouble breathing. She was also symptomatic for sepsis and needed treatment immediately, so the staff started her on IV fluids and antibiotics. Sarah, however, believed that her son had died because she brought him to the hospital, that it was the hospital itself, in essence, that killed him. So she took her daughter home, refusing further treatment. We could not force her to stay, but it seemed very unlikely that the little girl would survive without the care we could offer.

For generations, long before MSF arrived on the scene, people in and around Aweil went to traditional healers for medical care. This is the case in many countries where MSF works and Sarah went to one with her daughter after leaving our hospital. Luckily for all, the healer she visited knew the limits of his abilities. He advised Sarah to come back to us and our facility, so we could treat her little girl. A few days later, she returned.

The main issue in Sarah's case was that she simply did not know that she needed to feed her babies at night. Babies' stomachs are very small and they can't hold enough food to last eight hours. They need to be fed constantly.

Feeding can be its own issue, however. Breastfeeding is the best way to nourish a baby and a mother's milk helps the child build immunity against diseases. It contains antibodies and other agents that can prevent diarrhea, which can cause a baby to become dangerously underweight. This, too, needs to be explained in many cases, and some mothers need to be convinced that it's true. We heard some mothers say that the milk of a cow or a goat is better for a baby, when it decidedly is not.

Even if they are convinced, some mothers simply could not produce enough breast milk. They were malnourished themselves, or not drinking enough water. These mothers needed treatment before they'd be capable of producing enough milk for their babies.

Once Sarah began to trust us and the care we were providing, she followed all of our instructions on hygiene and feeding. While our staff administered antibiotics and oxygen to the baby, Sarah fed her daughter through the night. She bathed her during morning bath time and washed her linens every day. Our staff trained her to use a breast-pump, which encourages lactation, too.

The little girl got better. When Sarah brought her back for her three-month check up, just before I left the project, she was a normal, healthy child.

It feels odd to call an instance when only one twin survived a success story, but in this context it was. Given the hardships that babies in Aweil face, we were thrilled every time a newborn recovered from potentially fatal circumstances and began exhibiting the signs we hoped to see. This was partly because we knew how many other stories don't end as well.

Babies born early or small in under-resourced settings are particularly hard-pressed to get through their early days unscarred. Due to the fragile physiology of newborns, efforts to save their lives can damage their fragile ears or eyes and cause deafness or blindness—as in Deng Deng's case. They are also susceptible to bleeding in their brains. Staff have to make choices based on the resources at their disposal, and after saving the mother's life (because without their mother, her other children are far more likely to die), the foremost priority is saving a newborn's life.

There was a positive outcome for Sarah's daughter after her mother learned what her baby needed and provided it. The baby also survived because our staff at the hospital, while not neonatal specialists, were well trained and knew what to do for a sick newborn. This underscores how important it is for MSF to prepare, through continual training, the people working in its programs for the realities of what they are going to face, even if it's outside the realm of their previous experience.

In Aweil and other MSF facilities, midwives have first contact with the baby. They must assess the baby's breathing and if need be, start resuscitation and call for assistance. Midwives are also trained to check for hypoglycemia, hypothermia, and sepsis and to treat these complications if they arise. Nurses and nurse aides in Aweil were trained to advise mothers about feeding and how to use a breast pump if necessary to give milk on a regular basis. These are skills that may well fall outside the core training midwives, doctors, OBGYNs, nurses, and aides have had, skills they must learn. It's a function of necessity: in under-resourced areas neonatal units are rare, so staff need to be ready to go beyond the strict parameters of their profession. Midwives, for example, also need to learn to monitor and treat newborns for longer than a few hours after birth, and staff treating mothers post-partum should be trained in neonatal care as well.

And it's not just the skills; a certain attitude is needed to work in environments like these. Staff need to be ready to work with tiny little beings that seem extremely delicate. They must be comfortable working in situations where the stakes are, quite literally, life and death.

In our training in Aweil, we repeated the same things over and over and over again, drilling into our staff a set of simple, clear-cut protocols they should follow in every situation—if a baby is not breathing, for instance, or if a baby is hypothermic. MSF projects don't have the supplies, the equipment or the space of neonatal units in Paris, Tokyo, or New York, but our teams can still provide high-quality care by being consistent, thorough, and observant.

A real life example: in 2013, a young mother brought in two-day-old Joseph, whom she had given birth to at home. It was the mother's third pregnancy. Her first two babies had died and she was very worried it was about to happen again, especially because Joseph was not taking in much milk from her breast.

Our staff quickly saw that the baby was hypothermic and took him straight into our neonatal unit to warm him. The unit as a whole is kept very warm, but we have only one radiant warmer, which was occupied at the time by a preterm baby. We decided to switch the preterm baby to kangaroo care and put Joseph under the radiant warmer.

The nurse then inserted an IV line for him. Since hypoglycemia often follows hypothermia, we also tested his blood sugar level. It was low and we determined that he was in fact hypoglycemic. The staff had been trained to use the protocol for hypoglycemia and they immediately went into action.

Guidelines and protocols can make each stage and episode of treatment seem very linear, as if only one thing is happening at any given time, but that may not be the case. For example, the guidelines may say to test the blood sugar of a baby who weighs less than 5.5 pounds (2.5 kilograms) and administer intravenous fluids containing dextrose, a type of sugar. But there are times when a vein is difficult to locate, or, as with Joseph, the baby will have not one hypoglycemic episode but a series of them throughout the day and into the night. This is called rebounding. In these instances, the staff must figure out when they need to start over with the protocols and when they need to adapt.

Joseph was very sick. He needed to stay on antibiotics for several days, which was nerve-wracking for his mother. But he did recover, I'm happy to say. It was a challenge in a hospital with limited space, but we kept him as far away as possible from other babies in the unit so he didn't spread his infection onwards.

At MSF's project in Duékoué, Ivory Coast, our colleague found a novel solution to the same problem. She bought small plastic tubs to put the babies in, replacing the existing wooden boxes. To cover the babies they used sterile material from the operating theater instead of fabric the mothers brought in, which was not clean enough to limit the risk of infection.

After the staff in Duékoué implemented specific neonatal care protocols in 2012, the neonatal unit there saw a drop in newborn mortality even more dramatic than Aweil's. MSF had begun providing emergency care at Duékoué hospital in 2011, responding to an outbreak of violence in the area. Before the neonatal unit was installed in the hospital, newborns were being cared for in the open with other children and 80 percent of them did not survive. After MSF installed a tiny but functional neonatal nursery, we saw that figure come down to around 50 percent. Then, when the team had been trained to show mothers how to use breast pumps, to make sure babies were fed every three hours, and to adapt the environment further to reduce the risk of infection passed from one baby to another, as well as other straightforward skills, neonatal mortality fell to around 23 percent.

There are still more challenges to address, but this shows how seemingly small changes made a big difference in Duékoué, saving many more lives.

These initiatives are ongoing in more and more projects as MSF continues to implement integrated maternal and newborn care. For example, in Domeez camp in Iraqi Kurdistan, where around 60,000 Syrian refugees are now living, MSF opened a maternity center in August 2014. It offers complete maternal and newborn care from ANC to postnatal consultations.

MSF believes that integrating maternal and newborn care and providing comprehensive service are the best ways to lower neonatal deaths and to give babies who survive a better chance at long-term health, while keeping their mothers alive and healthy. All MSF maternity staff members are therefore being trained to improve basic newborn care and provide mothers with the information they need to keep their babies alive and healthy. There are limitations to what MSF can do, but we have already seen in places like Aweil and Duékoué that simple solutions can go a long way to saving lives.

[i] UNICEF, WHO, World Bank, UN, "Levels and Trends in Child Mortality 2013," World Health Organization, pg 1. 2014 http://www.who.int/maternal_child_adolescent/documents/levels_trends_child_mortality_2013/en/
[ii] Ibid.
[iii] Liu et al, "Global, regional, and national causes of child mortality: an updated systematic analysis for 2010 with time trends since 2000," The Lancet. June 9 2012. vol. 379, p. 2158-9. http://www.who.int/immunization/diseases/tetanus/lancet-2012-global-child-mortality.pdf

STORIES FROM PATIENTS AND STAFF

Wazmina, 35, Kabul, Afghanistan

"I brought my five-month-old baby here *[to MSF's Ahmad Shah Baba Hospital]* five days ago because she has been having fever and diarrhea. I have three sons and four daughters. All of them I delivered at home, assisted by my mother or sister.

This baby always cried. I took her to see the mullah. The mullah said she was fine but she was still crying. My sister-in-law lives in Ahmad Shah Baba and she knew MSF worked here with some foreign doctors and provided good quality care, so I came here. The doctor said the baby was malnourished and he asked me to stay here with her for two weeks so she could recover. I stayed, but I've been worried about my other children at home.

Two of my sons died when they were very small. One died when he was five months old and one when he was just 10 days. They had fever and diarrhea. We didn't know what was wrong with them.

When we took the five-month-old to another public hospital in Kabul, the doctor said it was too late. He died in the hospital. There is no private doctor or government clinic in our village. The closest place we can go is to the bazaar in Kapisa, 30 minutes by foot. It took us three hours to arrive here by car. The road is not good.

We don't always go to see a doctor when we are sick. Sometimes there is a conflict between the armed opposition and the government. There have been shootings in the village.

Sometimes we don't have the money to pay for medical care. Then we just stay home and rest. We borrowed money from people in the village for transport to come here, 7,000 afghanis [$121].

My husband works as a shopkeeper. We are poor. We don't have money. Usually we pay 600 afghanis [$10] to see a private doctor in Kapisa and another 50-150 afghanis [$0.87 to $2.60] for the medicines. I am glad that Ahmad Shah Baba Hospital is free of charge.

The women in our village all deliver at home. If they have complications, they go to Kapisa, but the doctors are not good. I heard some women died during delivery. Sometimes babies have died. There are a lot of stories like these."

Joyce, 27, mother of seven, Kibera, Kenya

"I did not even know I had twins in me. When I arrived at the MSF clinic, I was well received and taken to the labor ward. I was in labor for a few hours and it was time to deliver. My first twin came out all right but the second one got stuck inside me. How I wished I had come for regular visits at the clinic because this problem could have been identified much earlier.

Because I did not have the money for a Caesarean section, I was scared about what would happen. MSF was able to provide for the surgical procedures I had to undergo as well as the after-care. I could not otherwise have afforded these trips or the treatment. At this hospital, I went through a Caesarean birth for my first time ever. There were complications and by the time I left the hospital I had had four surgeries. I felt weak, sick and in pain. My children were underweight. Each weighed 1.6 kilograms (3.5 pounds). I was shocked—all my other children had been okay. My twins were put in an incubator for two weeks.

In my condition after the surgeries, the Government of Kenya social services intervened and took my twins to a children's home—I could not take care of them. They are now seven months old, and I have been able to save some money to go see them once. I am hoping I will work hard and be in a better financial position to take them back, though I am happy that I received such help when I was not in a position to protect and provide for them. I am just very grateful that I am alive and so are my children. I have seen many women here in the slums lose their babies during deliveries or after, and sometimes when they are a little older they die of malaria and hygiene-related diseases.

Kibera is a poor neighborhood. In such an environment, I make sure I am clean enough and try to feed my family a balanced diet when I have the money. Cleanliness is difficult though. Hygiene starts with water, and we have to buy water and food and this becomes a challenge. I do not have a job and I rely on washing people's clothes to make a living for myself and my children, so whatever I get, I have to spend wisely, knowing I might not get work tomorrow. This is very stressful and difficult especially as I am raising my children alone."

Dr. Marianne Sutton, pediatrician with MSF, Ivory Coast

"The situation *[in Duékoué hospital, Ivory Coast, during the fighting in 2011]* was chaotic at the beginning, as there had been so many other needs in the hospital. But women still give birth, conflict or not.

We knew we could implement some simple things that would help reduce the deaths of both mothers and newborns, the rates of which was enormous. My role was to help with the newborns.

The babies I saw dying in my first few weeks there were dying mainly of sepsis. They would get an infection, become pale, and then stop breathing. It was terrible to see all these babies dying.

When I arrived, we established a neonatal unit with standardized protocols, and we also encouraged exclusive breastfeeding, the sterilization of all the baby laundry, and the use of warm blankets. The mortality rate dropped drastically. It's important to note that the rate stayed down—this wasn't just a blip in the statistics.

Thanks to the Ivorian nurses' aides, who embraced teaching the mothers how to breastfeed or how to use the breast pump if the babies were not attaching to the breast, we were able to achieve this. The nurses' aides would encourage mothers to use the breast pump six to eight times per day, and then the milk was fed to the babies by syringe. This was all recorded in a flowchart. With the nurses' aides' devotion to the job and the enormous task of feeding 15 to 20 babies by syringe every three hours for a 12-hour shift, many babies' lives were saved."

Journal

What It Takes To Make A Difference:
An OBGYN's Journal in Sierra Leone
By Betty R. Raney, MD, OBGYN

My name is Betty Raney and I live in Charleston, South Carolina. I have worked as an obstetrician and gynecologist in the U.S. for 25 years, 22 of them in my hometown of Indianapolis. My first assignment with MSF was in Bo, Sierra Leone, for six months in 2012.

I know our team made a difference in Bo. By running a 24-hour, high-risk obstetric unit, and having a referral system to transport emergency patients from outlying villages and towns by ambulance to our facility—the Gondama Referral Center—MSF estimates the maternal death rate in Bo district decreased by 61 percent.

The maternal deaths were the hardest part of my mission; they were something I never thought I would experience in my career. With the first death, I was devastated for days. In the U.S. we can largely save young healthy women because we have every medical device, medication, and specialist at our fingertips. That was not the case in Sierra Leone. Whenever I was struggling with this, I talked to colleagues, and sometimes called home. Gradually, I accepted that I could not save everybody and it was not my fault. My efforts and concentration needed to go towards those I could save.

The following are excerpts from the journal I kept during my time in Bo.

June 1: Arrival

I'm writing in the car. Made it here late last night after an eight-hour flight to Brussels, then a six-hour flight to Lungi Airport, Sierra Leone. About an hour later I was on a boat to Freetown.

The MSF driver picked me up when I got off the boat and we drove to the MSF house. Even though it was dark, I was smacked in the face by the profound poverty. Rows and rows of homes that were nothing more than lean-tos made of sticks, tin, cloth—no bigger than one bedroom in my home and these were the homes of entire families.

I slept five hours and am now on a six-hour car trip to Bo. I skipped the briefings in Freetown today because they are so busy they need me in Bo right now.

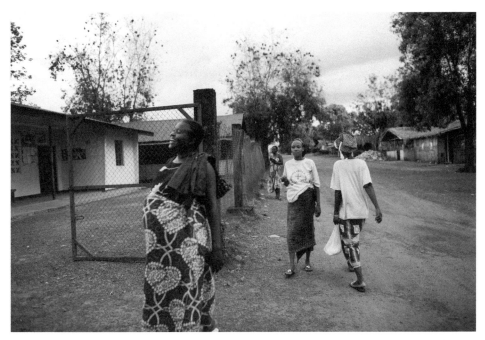

A pregnant patient waiting to give birth walks around outside the Gondama Referral Center in Bo, Sierra Leone. *Photo by Lynsey Addario/VII*

Whereas Freetown was dirty and noisy, the countryside is lush, tropical. It's amazing what the women can balance on their heads. Their clothing is so bright and beautiful. I don't know how it is so because none of the shanties have electricity, water, or even windows or doors.

I'm tired but I'm going to work.

June 2 My First Day
My OBGYN partner was evacuated yesterday due to possible exposure to a patient suspected of having Lassa fever[1]—the Lassa virus is endemic here.

One of my first patients had had a botched illegal abortion that extruded to the abdominal cavity. She was septic and very ill, only 16 years old. Note: She later died of infection.

There is lots of death here. According to the handover reports from other doctors, there have been one to four maternal deaths per month at the Gondama Referral Center. UNICEF reports that in 2012, 11.7 percent of infants born alive in Sierra Leone died and more than 18 percent of children under five died.[2]

June 3 How MSF Got Here
I just finished my rounds. I did a dilation and curettage (D&C)[3] for an incomplete spontaneous abortion or miscarriage and heavy bleeding. Then a Caesarean-section for a woman who had been in labor for three

---

[1] Lassa fever is an acute viral hemorrhagic illness caused by the Lassa virus.
[2] UNICEF, At A Glance: Sierra Leone, 2012, http://www.unicef.org/infobycountry/sierraleone_841.html
[3] D&C is a surgery done when a woman is having heavy vaginal bleeding from a miscarriage or another cause. It cleans out the uterine cavity, which is usually successful in stopping the bleeding.

days with a baby too large in relation to her pelvis to come out vaginal-ly—she had a placental abruption[4] and was bleeding.

Baby and mom are now doing well.

I learned that this hospital dates back to the war in Sierra Leone in the mid-nineties. MSF treated victims of the civil war, then refugees fleeing Liberia's civil war. It became Gondama Referral Center in 2007. Now it is here for the entire community and beyond as a measure to reduce maternal and child mortality.

June 4 Blood

After 24 hours on call, I am still wide awake due to the Lariam (meflo-quine hydrochloride) I've been taking to prevent malaria. My mind has been spinning with the day's activities—four C-sections for four live babies, one placental abruption, one hemorrhage/placenta previa,[5] one transverse lie,[6] one obstructed labor, and one D&C.

Any surgical patient here must have relatives to donate blood or she will not get blood during or after surgery if she needs it. If the lab has blood from another patient's donor, they won't let you have it because blood is so very scarce. If we take another patient's donated blood, she won't have blood when she may need it, which is unfair to her. In spite of this, it causes great anxiety in a doctor to know you have a patient who will die if she does not receive blood, and you see the unit you need sitting in front of you in the lab refrigerator.

---

[4] When the placenta peels away from the inner wall of the uterus before delivery, it can deprive the baby of oxygen and nutrients and cause heavy bleeding in the mother.
[5] When a baby's placenta partially or totally covers the mother's cervix—the opening between the uterus and the vagina. Placenta previa can cause severe bleeding before or during delivery.
[6] When a baby is positioned horizontally across the uterus, rather than vertically.

Note: I gradually learned how to get the lab guys to release blood to me in an emergency. I would promise to find other donors and they eventually learned that I was true to my word. It was a daily battle to find donors. We really needed a person to do just that, find donors, every day, all day long. Sometimes we recruited our mental health counselors for a couple of hours to do this for us.

June 5 Typical Injuries

Had a busy day, two interesting patients:

A 21-year-old who had a botched illegal abortion more than a week ago came in for pain. Her uterus was the size of a 4.5-month pregnancy, full of placental and fetal tissue. Someone had stuck an object into her to get her to abort, but the object never went into her cervix or uterus. Instead, it went from the vagina, through the vaginal wall, directly into the abdominal cavity. The damage was extensive. I tried to save the uterus but to no avail. I initially did a wedge resection, but then had to do a hysterectomy and removal of the right ovary.

A 14-year-old who delivered eight days ago had obstructed labor and her baby died. She now has a obstetric fistula—an opening between the vagina and the bladder—caused by the baby's head pressing hard against the pelvic bone for so long. She has also been having fevers and diarrhea. On rounds, her respiratory rate was 60 (normal is around 12) and blood pressure 60/40. Obviously, she is septic.[7] Is it endometritis or typhoid? Note: It turned out to be typhoid.[8] I started her on an antibiotic regimen. With typhoid, people get multiple tiny bowel per-

---

[7] Sepsis is an infection that has gone into the blood stream. Many people die from septic shock. The blood pressure becomes so low that blood does not reach all the critical organs, including the brain.
[8] Endometritis is inflammation or irritation of the lining of the uterus; typhoid is a life-threatening bacterial disease.

forations. We have no general surgeon on staff to take care of this. She may die tonight.

June 7 Foot Drop

The 14-year-old is no better, a little worse in terms of her fever and massive diarrhea. She does not have an acute abdomen. There is no cholera in the area.

I am seeing a lot of foot drop in these young women with obstructed labor. They are not able to pick up a foot as they walk, due to nerve damage. It happens when the baby is stuck low in the pelvis for so long that it presses on the nerves that go to the feet and the nerve dies off, permanently. They just live with it.

June 9 Unexpected Triplets

Today, I delivered triplets vaginally. I was unaware of the third baby until I was trying to find the placenta and felt his head. I hate delivering premature breeches—in the U.S., we always deliver these via C-section. Here, we do our best to avoid C-sections, because if a woman who has had a C-section gets pregnant again before her scar has healed and is unable to access emergency obstetric care, she is at great risk of dying. The first triplet was a breech—head was entrapped for around three minutes. The baby didn't make it. The second and third babies looked good but were much smaller. As healthy as they look, premature babies here have only a 20 percent chance of surviving the first 24 hours. If they make it home, they have a 30 percent risk of dying before age five.

June 11 Everyday Emergencies

Every day I see eclampsia—untreated high blood pressure that develops into seizures in pregnant women; ruptured ectopics—embryos that are implanted outside the uterus; obstructed labor; and retained placental and fetal tissue. A 19-year-old came in today who had taken large doses of "antibiotics" to abort. She had an incomplete abortion, needed D&C.

June 16 Illegal Abortions
I see patients daily with retained products from illegal abortions. A 14-year-old who was impregnated by her teacher and had an illegal abortion came in today. She had had a stick placed in her cervix for two days. She came in terribly infected—needed antibiotics, D&C.

I was confined to quarters for three days due to a 104°F/40°C fever. Haven't been that sick since I was 12 years old with dengue fever (I grew up in Thailand). First time I have ever missed work due to illness, except for a bike wreck. I'm homesick for family because I have had too much time on my hands.

June 19
Better now and back to work.

This truly is a difficult place for the people who live here. When you look around, it is beautiful, but it doesn't change what it is for people. Their lives are unimaginably difficult, every second of the day—never enough food, frequent illnesses that go untreated, sleeping in the dirt in an open shack at night.

June 20 Maternity Waiting Houses
Women here are most often pregnant 9 to 11 times and I have seen women have as many as 13 to 17 pregnancies. In spite of this they may have only two to six living children. There is a very high rate of still-birth and infant mortality. My assumption is that the high rate of still births is due to no prenatal care, poor nutrition, rampant hypertension in women, chronic severe anemia, malaria, and poor dental condition, which causes infections.

Most women give birth at home with a traditional birth attendant. Once a problem occurs, the pregnant woman still has miles to walk on foot from her village to our center. If she can't walk, family members may bring her on a motorbike—I saw it twice this morning. One man sits on the back of the motorbike and cradles the unconscious woman in his arms and she is wedged between him and the driver. It's amazing what people do with limited resources. But often they are too late—for both mother and child.

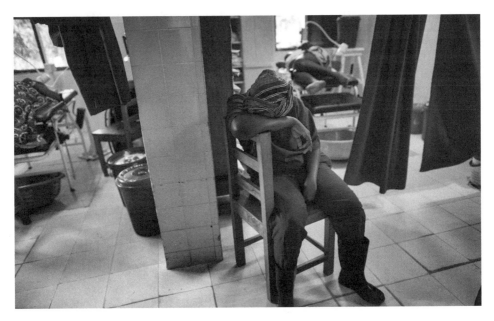

An exhausted health staff member takes a break. *Photo by Lynsey Addario/VII*

A major part of MSF's mission here is to reduce maternal and newborn mortality. We have constructed maternity waiting houses next to five outlying clinics in the area. When a woman starts labor, or even before labor, she can go to the waiting house with a caretaker and stay there. Patients and caretakers are fed, given beds, and they are provided with medical care.

The women then deliver in the clinics, which are staffed with midwives, and if there is a complication MSF has an ambulance at each clinic to transport the patient here to the Center for intervention. This saves thousands of lives, but the effort needs to be larger. More than 85 percent of women still deliver at home.

June 22 Female Genital Mutiliation

Today I sent home the 14-year-old patient who had undergone a dangerous abortion after being impregnated by her teacher. I treated her infection and gave her a contraceptive implant. She has about a 95 percent chance of infertility because her infection was severe enough to cause scarring and obstruction of her fallopian tubes.

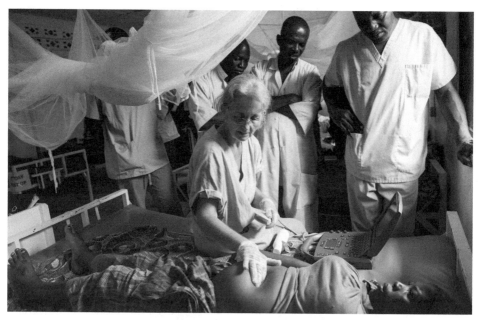

Dr. Raney and other medical staff discuss a patient's case. *Photo by Lynsey Addario/VII*

About 95 percent of women here have undergone female genital mutilation. In the form done here they cut off the clitoris and the labia minora. Women can suffer a lot of pain due to the scarring this causes. The procedure is performed by a person with no medical training in the community who may use the same blade on many girls. In Sierra Leone it happens around age 12, in other countries, like Sudan, it can happen earlier.

June 28 My First Maternal Death

I had the first maternal death of my 25-year career this week. This was a woman who came in with a dead baby due to a massive placental abruption. She had suffered a large amount of bleeding and was unstable from the second she entered our door. Her hemoglobin was 4.5 (a normal hemoglobin here is 6 or 7). Once she delivered, she was in disseminated intravascular coagulation (DIC), meaning all the clotting factors in the blood were used up. I worried about an undiagnosed uterine rupture as the uterus wasn't firming up. We kept losing blood pressure on her. She was transfused. I needed to do a hysterectomy.

When we finally got a blood pressure of 60/40 I did suprecervical hysterectomy (leaving the cervix in place) and filled her abdomen with packs. She got a total of five units of blood—no one here ever has the luxury of five units of blood. She lived about three hours post-op, but we had no way to reverse her DIC. Her bed was full of watery candy-colored blood when she died.

In talking to the other OBGYNs, I learned they also had never had a maternal death in their extensive careers until they worked in Sierra Leone. We have about one per week, sometimes up to seven per month. That is life as a woman in this part of Africa. This patient had six children at home. Her name was Betty. She was 36 years old. That day, every baby that came into my labor and delivery was dead ... every single one.

July 2 14-Year-Olds Aren't Supposed to Have Babies

Fatmata is the patient with typhoid I wrote about last month. She is a small girl, around 14 years old. She came to the Gondoma Referral Center with a dead baby and a ruptured uterus. She had surgery, then for two weeks was very sick with typhoid and almost died.

As a result of her obstructed labor she now has both a vesico-vaginal fistula—an opening between the vagina and the bladder—and a ure-thral-vaginal fistula—an opening between the vagina and the urethra. She walks around all day leaking urine. They do not have pads in the hospital, so she just leaks. I buy her bags of pads from the mini-mart but they go fast; she needs cases of them.

Not only that, she has severe pain in her right foot and right foot drop from the baby having compressed the nerves against her pelvic brim. Yesterday she was crying and moaning the pain was so severe. I started her on steroids and an analgesic and she is better today and walking a little easier. All of this—the fistula with urine leaking and the foot drop, which is permanent—is because 14-year-olds are not supposed to have babies.

Fatmata will soon be transferred to the West Africa Fistula Founda-tion extension at Bo Government Hospital. There is a surgeon from Texas who comes once a year to repair women's fistulas. I don't know if Fatmata's can be repaired because it involves a large portion of her urethra. It is a cruel thing for nature to allow fertility before it allows the body to be able to carry a baby without destroying it.

July 21 Against All Odds
Yesterday, a woman arrived in septic shock and DIC.[9] She would have arrived two hours earlier, but the ambulance at the clinic in Kenema had no fuel. If she had arrived a few minutes later she would have died. This woman had been having pain for about a month. After perform-ing a laparotomy[10] on her I determined that she had had a ruptured pregnancy in her fallopian tube, which occurred about a month ago.

---

[9] Disseminated intravascular coagulation (DIC), in which excessive blood clotting leads to the inability of the body to clot the blood at all.
[10] An incision through the abdominal wall to gain access to the abdominal cavity.

The pregnancy was expelled from the tube and the placenta then implanted on the right pelvic sidewall. It was approximately a 10-week pregnancy growing in her pelvis. Most women do not survive this type of thing, but she is doing well. We are down one person so I am on call every other day for a while—28 hours on, 20 hours off until a replacement arrives in a week or so. Only the other OBGYN and I seem to think this schedule is a problem.

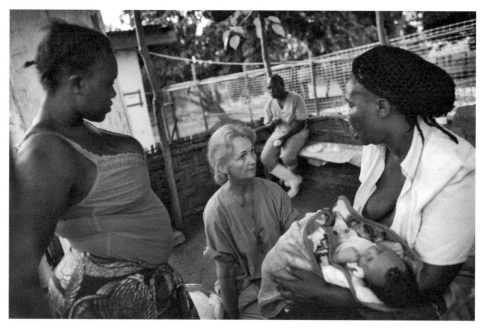

Dr. Raney speaks with a patient's relatives. *Photo by Lynsey Addario/VII*

A woman walked in with her baby's head presenting. It was a dead fetus and its head had been out for over 12 hours. The baby's shoulder was stuck; I relieved it and delivered the baby. It took me about 90 seconds. The patient was so grateful. The baby looked perfect and full term, but was dead.

I also did a C-section on a woman who came in with her baby's arm presenting. I've had three such presentations all in the same day here. In the U.S., I have seen it once in 25 years.

We see foot presentations every day—as well as eclampsia (seizures rom untreated high blood pressure), retained placental and fetal tissue, obstructed labor, and ruptured ectoptics (fetuses implanted in the fallopian tube).

July 25 A Miracle

There are small glimmers of hope here at times. A woman in septic shock who was stuck in Kenema for two hours for lack of fuel is alive and I think she will make it. This is very unusual in her circumstances and our chief health officer calls it "a truly miraculous case." These are the exact words he used when he and I went to the blood bank yesterday morning to beg for one more unit of blood for her. Her hemoglobin is still 4.6, which will not allow her to heal.

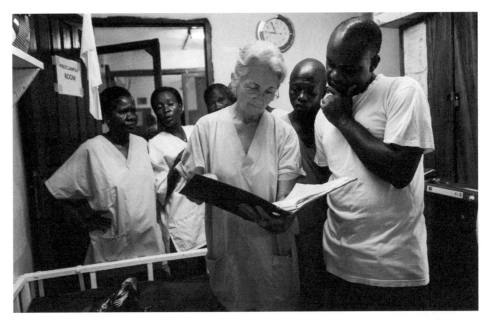

Dr. Raney conducts rounds with other medical staff at Gondama Referral Center. *Photo by Lynsey Addario/VII*

July 27 When the Pharmacy Is Closed

Except for Gondoma Referral Center, the hospitals in Sierra Leone do not have drugs or supplies such as bandages. If a patient goes to a hospital for a problem, the family is given a list of meds and supplies to go out and buy at the pharmacy for the patient. The pharmacies close at 9 p.m. Many patients die at night because there is no access to drugs they may need immediately.

Foday is one of our anesthetists. His 36-year-old brother died of a hypertensive crisis last week because he arrived at the hospital at night, and there were no drugs.

The other issue is payment. If the patient doesn't have the cash up front to pay for the surgery or treatment, the staff will watch the patient die of a ruptured uterus or ruptured appendix or whatever other ailment they have.

August 5 Eclampsia

Two days ago as I was finishing my shift at 7 a.m., the ambulance rolled in with a 17-year-old pregnant girl in a coma. At 10 a.m. the previous day she had had a seizure at home in her village. Her family placed her on a cloth stretcher and walked her to the nearest health center, which was a 20-hour walk. She was then put in an ambulance for a four-and-a-half hour drive over rough road, where her mother delivered the baby during transit.

When she arrived she had so much facial and neck edema (swelling) that her face and neck just blended in with her shoulders. She was stridorous, producing a high-pitched sound, due to swelling of her airway. Her blood pressure was high and she had protein in her urine, all the symptoms of severe, life-threatening eclampsia. We put a plastic syringe between her teeth so she would quit biting her tongue and started her on phenobarb, the only anti-epileptic med we have.

August 10

She is improving each day. The baby is fine. All in all a rough day for a 17-year-old.

August 19 Why Am I Here?

It was a terrible night. I feel like a boat that leaves nothing but death in its wake. I delivered 32-week twins by C-section three days ago. They were both transverse lie, lying sideways across the mother's abdomen. The second one died today, the first one yesterday.

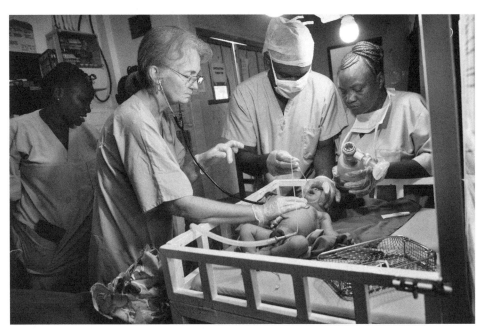

Medical staff with Dr. Raney treat a newborn baby. *Photo by Lynsey Addario/VII*

A 19-year-old girl came in with cephalopelvic disproportion (CPD)— she had pushed so long and so hard at home, that the baby's head had molded to try to fit through the birth canal. The baby was too far down at the time of the C-section, so I pushed it up before starting and the nurse pushed it up during the operation, but my hand still would not fit down past her pubic bone. With a head-down C-section we usually scoop the baby's head to pull it through the incision, but in this case it was not possible. So I extended the uterine incision and had to find the feet to pull the baby out as only the head and feet can fit through a small incision. This was the first time I had delivered a head-down baby feet first. The baby died, two hours after delivery.

August 24 Resilience

About 12 days ago, the 17-year-old who arrived in a coma started to walk with a walker and her seizures were lessening, but she had urinary retention and was unable to go to the bathroom. Her walking continued to improve every day and she had no foot drop. Today she went home on meds for chronic hypertension only. This woman undoubtedly had a stroke, followed by an amazing recovery. The healing properties of the body plus the resilience of women here amaze me.

August 27 A Child Victim of Rape

Last night I saw an eight-year-old sexual assault victim. Most of the sexual assaults here are on female children under the age of ten, all the way down to one-year-olds. This child was held by a man at knifepoint. He perforated through her vagina into her abdominal cavity. Her perineum was torn wide open and her rectal opening was damaged. She was having heavy vaginal bleeding. I have treated her for all sexually transmitted diseases and she is being prophylaxed for HIV. She has received tetanus and hep B vaccines. I'll be able to repair her injuries.

September 12 Another Child Victim of Rape

The eight-year-old who was raped went home today. She is running, laughing, and singing and seems to be a totally different child. I spoke to my partner who is on call tonight. She is tending to a rape victim who is one year, eight months old. She was raped by her father and is bleeding.

Lots of good things happen at our hospital, too. Lots of lives saved. Still lots to be done.

October 12 One Crisis After Another
Rough 24 hours on call. I started rounds at 8:15 a.m. and had 25 patients to see. The labor room was full and stayed full for the entire 24 hours.

My first patient was a C-section on a woman with two prior C-sections. It took two hours as the scar tissue from the previous operations was so bad.

Then I ran out to do a vacuum delivery on a woman who was screaming and would not push. Then I had a second C-section on a woman with obstructed labor whose vulva was swollen to the size of a large grapefruit. I then came out to stitch up a woman bleeding from an extensive vaginal laceration, which occurred at a clinic during delivery.

Now there was a third C-section to do on a patient whose cervix was so swollen that there was no way a baby could come through. Her C-section was as difficult as the first one of the day.

After I finished rounds I delivered a VBAC—a vaginal birth for a woman who had previously had a Caesarean. Her previous baby had died and this one was dead by the time she arrived at the hospital.

The entire 24-hour shift continued this way and I finally emptied the labor room at 7:30 the next morning, just in time to turn it over to my partner and to decide that I am in no hurry to come back!

November 17 Leaving Soon

I leave here in a week. It doesn't seem possible I have been here for six months. I don't feel quite ready to leave, as all the OBGYNs are brand new and don't know the ins and outs of the department yet. I guess it will sort itself out. Almost all the expats who were here when I arrived are gone. I will miss this place and the people here.

Our mission at the Gondoma Referral Center has expanded—there are now 28 expats instead of 23. Maternal mortality in Sierra Leone is 1 in 8, but in the Bo catchment area we have reduced the rate to better than even odds.

I've felt so needed and useful here, as though the little bit of time that I gave made a big difference in my patients' lives. I've learned a great deal, and I've received more than I've given. Our project is a very worthwhile effort.

Note: During the peak of the Ebola outbreak in West Africa in late 2014, the Gondoma Referral Center was closed as patients and staff could not be guaranteed safety. As of early 2015, this had left a huge gap in health care for women in Bo.

The Contributors

Martina Bacigalupo was born in 1978 in Genoa, Italy. After studying literature and philosophy in Italy, she studied photography at the London College of Communication. In 2007 she moved to Burundi, East Africa, where she continues to work as a freelance photographer, often in collaboration with international NGOs [among others: Human Rights Watch, Amnesty International, Doctors Without Borders/Médecins Sans Frontières (MSF), and Handicap International]. Her work has been published on the New York Times, Sunday Times Magazine, Le Monde, Vanity Fair, Esquire, Liberation, Internazionale, and has been shown in several international venues, including PARIS PHOTO 2013, UNSEEN, Amsterdam 2014, and AIPAD New York 2014. She won the Canon Female Photojournalist Award in 2010 and the Fnac Award for photographic creation in 2011. She is member of AGENCE VU in Paris and is represented by Grimaldi Gavin Gallery in London.

Dr. Helen Bygrave trained at Cambridge University and University College London School of Medicine, qualifying as a general practitioner in 1995. Since 2005, she has worked for MSF, supporting HIV/TB programs across Africa and Asia. She currently works as one of MSF's HIV/TB advisors in the Southern Africa Medical Unit. One of her major focuses has been supporting the field implementation of Prevention of Mother to Child HIV Transmission (PMTCT) programs, including operationalizing PMTCT B+.

Eva de Plecker is a midwife. She completed the International Course on Planning and Management of Reproductive Health Programs at Prince Leopold Institute of Tropical Medicine in Antwerp in 2008. She began working for MSF in 2004 in Rwanda, Ethiopia, Papua (Indonesia), Zimbabwe, Democratic Republic of Congo, and Haiti. From 2010

240

to 2011 she worked as sexual and reproductive health referrent and currently is an advisor for sexual and reproductive health at MSF-Belgium.

Dr. Séverine Caluwaerts qualified as a gynecologist-obstetrician in 2007 in Belgium, her home country. During her residency she spent one year in South Africa where she cared for a large population of HIV-positive women. After finishing her specialization, she did a six-month tropical medicine course and in 2008 went to work with MSF in Sierra Leone, to which she has returned several times. She has also worked in Democratic Republic of Congo, Niger, Burundi, Pakistan, and Afghanistan in MSF's maternal health projects. When she is not on mission, she works with HIV-positive pregnant women in Belgium and is involved in teaching medical students and midwives. She is also one of the referent gynecologists for MSF.

Joanne Cyr, Psy.D., is a clinical health psychologist and advisor on patient support, education & counseling (PSEC) for MSF-Switzerland. She also works for MSF as a flying specialist/PSEC implementer, travelling to different MSF projects to aid in strategic planning, evaluation of program activities, and training and coaching teams to strengthen a patient-centered approach to care in health structures and communities. She has worked with MSF since 2010, involved in training, mentoring and implementation of activities to support Prevention of Mother to Child HIV Transmission (PMTCT), adherence counseling by HIV/TB expert patients, and community models of sensitization, testing and counseling on HIV and TB.

Patrick Farrell has been a photographer with The Miami Herald since 1987. He is the recipient of the 2009 Pulitzer Prize for Breaking News Photography—awarded for his photographs of the devastation in Haiti caused by a particularly brutal hurricane season. Farrell has documented three decades of major news events, both locally and abroad, including the 1989 race riots in Miami's Overtown neighborhood, political and civil unrest in Haiti during the country's 1994 military rule, Hurricane Andrew's 1992 path of destruction in South Florida, the 1999 earthquake in Turkey, the Columbine High School massacre, and childhood poverty in the Americas. He has won numerous awards for his coverage of Haiti, including a Feature Photography Award in 2008 from the Overseas Press Club, two first place awards from Pictures of the Year International (also in 2008), and the first place 2009 National Headliner Award for Photo Essay. Farrell has been named Region Six Photographer of the Year twice by the National Press Photographers Association. He is an adjunct professor of photography at Florida International University, where he is helping develop a photojournalism program for the FIU School of Journalism and Mass Communications. Born in Miami, he graduated from the University of Miami in 1981. Farrell is married to Miami-based journalist Jodi Mailander Farrell and they have two young daughters.

Kate Geraghty started work as a photographer in 1997 and has been a staff photographer with the Sydney Morning Herald since 2001. In that time she has covered the 2002 Bali bombings, the 2003 invasion of Iraq, South Asian Tsunami, 2006 war in Lebanon, humanitarian crisis in the DRC, South Sudan's historical referendum vote for independence, Gaza flotilla attack in 2010, Afghanistan and Papua New Guinea in 2013. In 2014, Kate covered life under sanctions in Iran, the Crimea crisis, the war in East Ukraine including the MH17 downing, and has just returned from covering the war against ISIS in Iraq. She was recently awarded 2013 Nikon Walkley Press Photographer of the Year, Australia.

Olivia Hill is a reproductive and sexual health referent in the medical department of MSF-Spain. She is a nurse and midwife with a specialization in tropical diseases and holds a masters degree in Sexual and

Reproductive Health Research from the London School of Hygiene & Tropical Medicine. She began working with Action Against Hunger in 1998, traveling to Afghanistan, Sudan, and Cambodia, and joined MSF in 2000 where she supported sexual and reproductive health activities in Eritrea, Sierra Leone, Somalia and Colombia. She has contributed to MSF's field research through evaluations of rapid diagnostic tests for malaria in Colombia, investigating the gap between the use of antenatal and delivery services in northern Uganda, and documenting the sexual and reproductive health consequences for victims of trafficking in Morocco. In addition, she represents MSF as an active member of the Interagency Working group (IAWG) on reproductive health in crisis and is a contributing author to the 2010 IAWG field manual.

Kristin Hooper, a registered nurse, has worked in a variety of health care settings. Starting out working in an adult cardiac intensive care unit (ICU), she discovered pediatrics by chance. Over the last eight years, she has worked in a neonatal ICU, a pediatric ICU, in pediatric oncology, and in several adult and pediatric emergency rooms at home in the United States and abroad. She worked with MSF for five months in Aweil, South Sudan, with a focus on pediatrics. Currently, Hooper works as a pediatric flight nurse at Oregon Health and Science University and is finishing a graduate degree in Family Practice Nursing.

Dr. Michiel Lekkerkerker qualified as a MD in 1983, and received additional training in emergency surgery, obstetrics, radiology, and family medicine in Holland, the Netherlands Antilles, and South Africa. Between 1985 and 1995 he worked mainly in Africa as a district health manager with heavy clinical duties. He has vast experience in war surgery and emergency obstetrics in resource-poor settings. After a brief stint as general practitioner in Holland, he started working for MSF-Holland in 1999 as a health advisor supporting MSF projects in various countries. He has been the surgical advisor for MSF-Holland for eight years. He is also a reproductive health advisor and a member of MSF's intersectional working group on sexual and reproductive health. He has a particular interest in the issue of obstetric fistula and he introduced a model of care for women living with fistulas in MSF-Holland.

Meinie Nicolai first worked with MSF in 1992, as a supervising nurse in Liberia. She has since gained a decade of field experience in Angola, the Democratic Republic of the Congo, Ethiopia, Rwanda, Somalia and South Sudan. Nicolai then returned to her native Netherlands to coordinate national network on sexual and reproductive health and AIDS between 2002 and 2003, but her involvement with MSF continued and she became a board member of the Belgian association. In 2004, she became director of operations in the Brussels office until October 2010 when she was elected president of both MSF-Belgium and MSF's operational directorate in Brussels.

Pamela A. Onango is a registered nurse-midwife from Kenya . Among other assignments, she has supervised mobile clinics and networked with traditional birth attendants in South Sudan, helped implement an Option B+ Prevention of Mother to Child HIV Transmission (PMTCT) pilot program in Swaziland, and set up a reproductive health department in an emergency project for internally displaced people in South Sudan. Before joining MSF in 2009, she worked with Kenya's Ministry of Health for 14 years.

Dr. Nicolas Peyraud, MD, is a pediatrics specialist and serves as Pediatric Advisor for MSF-Switzerland. After completing his training in Switzerland he joined MSF in 2009 as a pediatrician, working at an MSF project in Niger. In 2010 he developed a training plan designed to improve the quality of medical care for malnutrition with a focus on high-level hospital care for malnourished children. He then implemented the training for MSF field staff in Zinder, Niger, and in Dadaab, Kenya. He joined the MSF-Australia Project Unit in 2011 as a pediatric advisor, focusing on hospital care for sick newborns and sick children. He provides supervision remotely and in the field for MSF projects in countries including South Sudan, Central African Republic (CAR), and Jordan.

Aerlyn Pfeil is a certified professional midwife from Portland, Oregon. In 2011, after working as a home birth midwife, she joined MSF and went on to work in South Sudan, Haiti, Senegal, the Somali region of Ethiopia, and Papua New Guinea. In addition to performing clinical maternal health work, she has trained midwives and community health workers and treated survivors of sexual violence. Pfeil has also trained MSF staff on gender issues and the delivery of medical and psychological care for sexual violence survivors. In 2014, she served as medical team leader for MSF's treatment and training program for survivors of family and sexual violence in Papua New Guinea.

Debbie Price is a certified nurse-midwife and has been working with MSF since 1998. Her field experience includes serving as a medical coordinator in Democratic Republic of the Congo, Tajikistan, Pakistan, Sudan (Darfur), and Haiti. She has trained first-time medical coordinators and has been a member of the MSF emergency team. Price has also conducted program project evaluations for MSF in Cambodia and Russia (North Caucasus). She holds a Doctor of Public Health degree and her academic work has been focused on reproductive health in emergency settings. She is now based in the MSF-Holland office where she serves as the reproductive health specialist advisor for ten projects, and as coordinator of medical specialists for fifteen office staff.

Dr. Betty Raney earned her medical degree from Indiana University Medical School. She completed her residency in obstetrics and gynecology at Methodist Hospital in Indianapolis, Indiana in 1990, and has been actively practicing since that time. She spent six months as a practicing obstetrician and gynecologist with MSF in Gondama, Sierra Leone in 2012.

Nele Segers, studied midwifery and tropical medicine and earned her Masters degree in Nursing and Midwifery Sciences as well as her teaching degree in Belgium. She joined MSF in 2007, working as a midwife first in Sierra Leone, then in Chad, Democratic Republic of Congo, Central African Republic, Afghanistan, Haiti, Ethiopia and South Sudan. In 2012 Segers started work for a year as a mentor for MSF midwives on their first assignment with MSF-Spain in Ethiopia, Yemen, and Syria, and other countries. After working for a short period at the University Hospital of Brussels, she returned to Central African Republic in 2014 as coordinator for an MSF maternity project. Segers was trained as a global ALSO (Advanced Life Support in Obstetrics) course instructor and has assisted in training staff in Denmark, Nairobi and India. She has also trained staff on treatment for sexual violence victims in Yemen and Nairobi.

Catrin Schulte-Hillen began working with MSF in 1989 as a midwife, going on to serve as a project coordinator and project manager in conflict and post-conflict contexts in Africa, Latin America, and the Balkans. Before becoming MSF's reproductive health and sexual violence care working group leader, Schulte-Hillen was program director for MSF-USA and worked for several years as a health advisor and consultant on a number of specific assignments and evaluations for MSF and for other NGOs and the European Commission. As working group leader, Schulte-Hillen contributes to defining MSF's vision, medical policies, and strategies, and to improve assistance in the areas of reproductive health and sexual violence care. She is a licensed midwife and holds a Masters of Public Health, a license in applied epidemiology and statistics, and a degree in business administration.

Rebecca Singer is a doctorally prepared nurse with over a decade of experience in humanitarian response and development work. She spent nearly five years with MSF focusing on providing services to survivors of sexual and family violence in Liberia, Kenya, Chad, DRC, Zimbabwe and Papua New Guinea. She also worked with survivors of torture who had immigrated to the United States, ensuring that they had adequate health care services. Following her tenure with MSF, Rebecca has worked with several development organizations dedicated to improving the quality of life of coffee farmers. She is currently the executive director of Coffee Kids. Prior to becoming a nurse, she worked in community relations and as a communications manager for a membership organization. These experiences have shaped her philosophy that embraces both direct patient care and advocacy with a community approach.

Sydelle Willow Smith is a freelance photographer/filmmaker from Johannesburg, South Africa, now based in Cape Town. She is keenly interested in the subject of migration. Her 2014 public art project Soft Walls featured photos that sought to deal with convivial relationships between migrated African nationals and South Africans. Smith's short film Vecinos (Neighbours), 2013, was completed as part of a residency at Jiwar, Creation and Society based in Gracia, Barcelona, funded by The Africa Centre and the Spanish Embassy of South Africa. Of this project, where she used video, documentary and participatory photography, Smith says: "I am intrigued by how people who are a minority, such as African 'migrants' in Barcelona, navigate the city. What is their experience of it? What happens after one survives the treacherous crossing by boat, or how has the experience changed after living here for twenty years…" Smith is currently completing her Masters of Science in African Studies at Oxford University through St. Antony's College.

Ann Van Haver studied midwifery at Artevelde Hogeschool in Gent, Belgium, completing her internship in two Ugandan hospitals. After acquiring her undergraduate degree, she worked in a private hospital in Uganda, where she learned most of her technical skills. In 2006, she worked in the maternity and delivery room of a hospital in Brussels, where the majority of patients were immigrants, and took a course on tropical medicine for nurses and midwives in Antwerp. In 2007, Van Haver joined MSF, going on to work as a midwife in Liberia, South Sudan, Darfur, Central African Republic, Burundi, Pakistan and Afghanistan. She has also provided sexual and reproductive health (SRH) consultations, helped integrate Prevention of Mother to Child HIV Transmission (PMTCT) services into maternal care projects, assisted medical treatment for sexual violence, set up SRH activities, and, in Afghanistan, serving as a project's medical referrent. Central in all of her field work with MSF has been the training and coaching of national staff. In 2013, Van Haver began working as a SRH mobile implementation officer for MSF-Belgium, supporting different MSF projects to offer quality SRH services, coaching field workers on their first assignments with MSF, and implementing new SRH activities.

The MSF Charter

Doctors Without Borders/Médecins Sans Frontières (MSF) is a private, international association. The association is made up mainly of doctors and health sector workers and is also open to all other professions which might help in achieving its aims. All of its members agree to honor the following principles:

•MSF provides assistance to populations in distress, to victims of natural or man-made disasters, and to victims of armed conflict. They do so irrespective of race, religion, creed, or political convictions.

•MSF observes neutrality and impartiality in the name of universal medical ethics and the right to humanitarian assistance and claims full and unhindered freedom in the exercise of its functions.

•Members undertake to respect their professional code of ethics and maintain complete independence from all political, economic, or religious powers.

•As volunteers, members understand the risks and dangers of the missions they carry out and make no claim for themselves or their assigns for any form of compensation other than that which the association might be able to afford them.

Learn more at doctorswithoutborders.org